Preface to Soutra

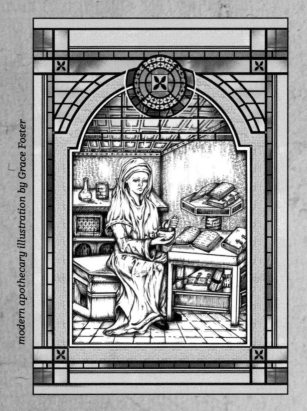

A modern perspective

A window on Medieval medicine

The drains at Soutra Monastery give up their herbal secrets

Including
a modern Macer translation by
Sarah Atkinson

Introduction
Jan Parkin

Illustrated by
R. A. Parkin

1150 ~ 2018

Preface to Soutra ~ A window on The Drains

This is a book about a medieval monastery whose existence is revealed only by the presence of a drain. A very special drain filled with medical waste and blood perfectly preserved in clay.

About twenty years ago I went to a weekend of lectures about Soutra run by Professor Brian Moffat - I was transfixed by his energy and enthusiasm for his subject; he has been excavating the drains and cellars at Soutra for over 30 years. For many years afterwards I used his SHARP (Soutra Hospital Archaeological Research Project) Practice books as a basis for my talks on herbal medicine - I seized any opportunity to mention Soutra and its drains! One day I decided to write to Brian and ask him if he had written the definitive book on Soutra.

He hadn't, but as my interest is primarily herbal I decided, with Brian's encouragement, to write a book about Soutra from a herbal perspective.

Here it is.

But, it wasn't quite that simple, I found it very difficult to decide where to start. It was only when I was outlining my problem to my friend Jan that I realised that I was talking to the right person - an English scholar with a passion for history - she helped me start the book by writing the introduction. Then we needed some illustrations - Jan's sister Ruth is a talented illustrator and an archaeologist, we had found someone to fill this gap. Finally it occurred to me that it would be amazing if I knew someone who understood how to put a book together - I was talking this through with my friend Sally when the penny dropped that this was her area of expertise. Not forgetting some early help from a very old friend Hayley, who suggested that 'flip books' always go down well (her son Glen was 7 at the time), which was skillfully brought to life by Ruth in her illustrations of the monk and his dog pulling up a mandrake root at the bottom right hand corner of the pages half way through the book.

You could say all this happened through happy accident or was it meant to be?

Sarah Atkinson
MNIMH dip. phyt.
Medical Herbalist
www.medicine-garden.com

Volume One
Sarah Atkinson

Sarah is a Medical Herbalist, she focuses on what we eat and drink combined with listening to people's life stories, which makes for a much more holistic approach to dis-ease.
www.medicine-garden.com

First published in 2018
By Sarah Atkinson
Orchard Head
Foxfield
Broughton-in-Furness
Cumbria LA20 6BT

Edited by Jan Parkin

Illustrations, linocuts and herb drawings by:
© R.A. Parkin; rydal3@aol.com

The facsimile pages found in this book are from a printed copy of Macer Floridus De Viribus Herbarum held at the British Library.
A full copy of an alternative printed version can be found on-line here:
www.e-rara.ch/gep_g/content/titleinfo/1752735

Designed & produced by Sally Bamber
www.sallybamber.com

Printed by Beam Reach Printing
www.beamreachuk.co.uk

Further copies of this book may be obtained from Sarah Atkinson
£18, email: sarah.atkinson4941@live.co.uk

ISBN 978-1-5272-2572-5

Contents

IX   Herbalists through time
and the Scottish Power Struggle 1107-1440 AD

XIII   A Window on Medieval Medicine

XX   A medieval monastery's approach to running an infirmary

1   **21st Century Modern Macer Translation**

2   **Contents of Macer herbs**

4   **Essential herbs**

121   **Spices**

138   **Not to be forgotten herbs**

XXVIII   Mandrake

XXXI   Soutra hospital research project excavations

XLIV   Bitter Vetch

XLVI   A history of medieval anaesthesia

XLVIII   Henbane

XLIX   Hemlock

LI   Poppy

LV   Ergot

LV   Juniper

LVI   Blood letting

LIX   Anthrax

LX   Extracts from John Skelton

LXIII   Soutra and Macer: a summary of health care

LXIV   Looking at the most common conditions mentioned

LXVIII   In conclusion

LXIX   Index of herbs; Latin, Medieval and Common names

LXXII   Glossary

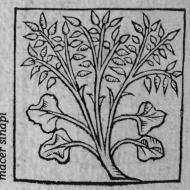

macer sinapi

Herbalists through time and the Scottish Power Struggle 1107-1440 AD

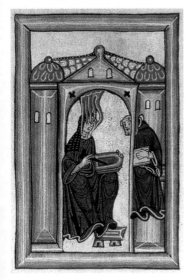

Hildegard von Bingen receiving divine inspiration, medieval manuscript

460 BC - 370 BC; Hippocrates, Considered to be the father of western medicine - his approach to illness was that he considered an imbalance of 'humours' caused ill health which could be healed by a change in diet or lifestyle rather than attributing illness to witchcraft or upsetting the gods - which was the thinking of the time. Quotes attributed to him - 'Let food be thy medicine and medicine be thy food' and 'walking is man's best medicine'.

129 AD - 216 AD; Galen, Claudius Galenus was a physician to the gladiators - only five gladiators died during his tenure as opposed to over 60 during his predecessors' time. He was a keen vivisectionist using pigs or primates which gave him great insights into the workings of the body as well as following Hippocrates principles. Galen promoted the idea of blood letting which was taken up enthusiastically in western medicine particularly during the middle ages. He was also a prolific author and is thought to have written over 10 million words, three million of which are still in existence - one of his most famous works is 'The Best Phsician is also a Philosopher'.

40 AD - 90 AD; Dioscorides, Pedanius Dioscorides was an army surgeon under the Roman emperor Nero - this gave him first hand experience of using herbs as medicine which he used to write De Materia Medica - this ran to five volumes covering 600 plants. This book has never been out of print and has been a reference book for physicians for nearly 2000 years.

23-79 AD; Pliny the Elder, wrote 'A Natural History', this ran to many volumes which he dedicated to Titus in 77 AD.

C10; Macer Floridus, although the first written copies still in existence were copied in C15 they were probably originally written in early C10.

C10; Medical School of Salerno established second half of the C10, at its height in 11-13th centuries eventually closing in 1812.

1098-1179; Hildegard Von Bingen wrote about plants and medicine in Liber Simplicus Medicinae comprising nine books in 1158.

1107 Alexander I becomes king of Scotland and rules until 1124. **1120** Foundation of the Monastery at Soutra. **1124** Alexander I dies and is succeeded by David I, his younger brother. **1138** The English defeat David I of Scotland who is fighting on behalf of Matilda, also known as Maud, daughter of Henry I of England. **1153** Malcolm IV 'The Maiden,' grandson of David becomes King of Scotland. **1165** William 'The Lion,' younger brother of Malcolm IV becomes King of Scotland. **1286** Alexander III king of Scotland dies and the throne descends to his granddaughter Margaret, the maid of Norway. **1290** Margaret dies leading to a bloody power struggle in Scotland. **1292** John Balliol rules Scotland on behalf of Edward I. **1296** Edward I deposes John Balliol. **1297** William Wallace leads the Scots to victory over the English at the battle of Cambuskenneth, a brief period of independence for the Scots. **1298** Edward I defeats William Wallace at the battle of Falkirk (the first documented use of the English long bow). **1305** The English capture and execute William Wallace. **1306** Scottish rebellion led by Robert the Bruce - he is crowned king of Scotland and ends a 10 year interregnum in Scotland. **1307** King Edward dies while on campaign against Robert the Bruce. **1314** After years of guerrilla warfare, Robert the Bruce defeats the English conclusively at Bannockburn. (The Bannockburn battle ground is within sight of Soutra Monastery). **1329** David II king of Scotland. Succeeds to the throne after his father Robert the Bruce dies. **1331** England at war with Scotland and Scotland's French allies. **1332** Edward Balliol son of John Balliol attempts to seize the Scottish throne with the help of the English. He is defeated. **1333** Edward III invades Scotland on Balliol's behalf and defeats the Scots at the battle of Halidon Hill. **1357** The Scots ransom David II from the English. **1371** Robert II, king of Scotland takes the Scottish throne. He rules until 1390 as the first Stuart monarch in Scotland. Richard II, with his uncle John of Gaunt, undertakes a military campaign in Scotland , this is unsuccessful. **1390** Robert III becomes king of Scotland.

1406; On the death of Robert III, James I becomes king of Scotland.

1437; James I dies and his son James II becomes King of Scotland.

1440; The inhabitants of Holy Trinity at Soutra move to Edinburgh to the current site of Waverley station.

1518; Master Martin the physician appears in the directory of medical practitioners. The only physician to be mentioned in Soutra's records.

1508-1568; William Turner wrote 'A New Herbal' in three parts between 1551 and 1568. The first herbal to be written in English, clearly describing the herbs.

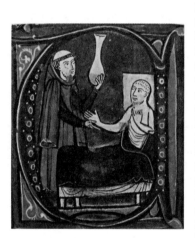

The Incredible Medical Interventions of the Monks of Soutra Aisle

http://www.ancient-origins.net/ancient-places-europe/incredible-medical-interventions-monks-soutra-aisle-003285 (Wikimedia Commons)

1567-1650; John Parkinson set up the Society of Apothecaries in 1617, became apothecary to James I. In 1629 he published the first book on gardening 'Paradisi in sole paradisius terrestris' or 'A Garden of all sorts of pleasant flowers which our English air will permit to be nourished up with a Kitchen Garden'.

1616-1654; Nicholas Culpepper wrote a translation of the Pharmacopeia of The College of Physicians from Latin into English called 'A Physical Directory' or a 'Translation of the London Dispensary' in 1649; through this book he challenged the monopoly of physicians and apothecaries by providing enough information for people to make up their own remedies.

1641-1712; Sir Robert Sibbald founded the Royal College of Physicians of Edinburgh and established Scotland's first physic garden. He wrote 'Scotia Illustrata' in 1641 an extensive work covering Scotland's flora and fauna.

1768; James Robertson made at least three tours of Scotland in the C18 recording the people and plants as he went. His most well documented travels were in 1768 when he described the harvesting and uses of bitter vetch or heath pea by 'the poor people'. He was a gardener at Edinburgh's Royal Physic garden.

1710-1790; William Cullen, Scottish Physician, initially apprenticed to a Glasgow surgeon-apothecary. He became an active member of the Royal College of Physicians of Edinburgh from 1756 until his death. He was particularly famous for his lectures on chemistry, materia medica, diagnosis and physiology.

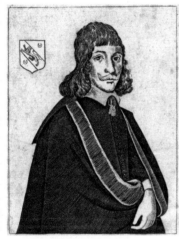

Nicholas Culpeper (1616-1654), English physician, herbalist and astrologer. In 1649, Culpeper translated the College of Physicians' Pharmacopoeia from Latin to English. The book included sections on the preparation and uses of drugs. This unauthorised translation was popular with the public but made him many enemies in the medical establishment who resented their loss of a monopoly on knowledge. Artwork from A Physical Directory (London, 1651).

Credit: Middle Temple Library / Science Photo Library

1769-1843; Albert Isaiah Coffin practised botanical medicine following the Thompsonian approach. (Both Dr. Coffin and Samuel Thompson were Americans and were particularly active before the civil war in America) Dr. Coffin came to England in 1839.

1805-1880; John Skelton, active around the same time as Dr. Coffin, set up a publication called The Botanic Record 1848 - 1852

1858-1941; Maude Grieve, wrote 'A Modern Herbal', helped to found the National Herb Growing Association.

1863; National Institute of Medical Herbalists founded.

1995; Thomas Bartram, wrote his Encyclopaedia of Herbal Medicine in 1995 and founded Gerard House.

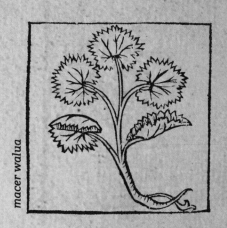

macer walua

A Window on Medieval Medicine

The drains at Soutra Monastery give up their Herbal Secrets

Introduction
Jan Parkin

Location

The sandstone ruins of Soutra Aisle lie a short distance within the Scottish borders, 2 miles southeast of Fala. They form the remains of the House of the Holy Trinity, once part of a large complex of buildings comprising a hospital and friary ; it was the highest monastic foundation in Great Britain at 1100 ft. In terms of modern roads it lies half a mile along the B6368 from its junction with the A68. In the High Middle Ages Soutra lay on the more evocatively named via Regia or royal way. This route connected the larger northern areas of Scotland with the important ecclesiastic sites of the Scottish borders. The via Regia formed part of the much larger Dere Street, a Roman road between Eboracum, (York) and Veluniate, (Borrowstounness), at the eastern limit of the Antonine Wall in Scotland. The name Dere Street was derived from the post- Roman Anglo-Saxon kingdom of Deira through which the first part of its route lay. The ideas that may suggest themselves upon hearing the words 'street' and 'royal way' probably need to be revised downwards. Following the destruction of the border abbeys in the Anglo-Scottish wars and during the Reformation of the Scottish Church the route fell into disrepair being used largely for driving herds of livestock from town to town and by groups of travellers brave enough to venture forth into the lawless border regions. Even in the heyday of Soutra this route would have resembled to the modern eye little more than a well-trodden track way. (Map on page XXXII)

Soutra and the Order of St Augustine

In its heyday the House of Holy Trinity at Soutra was one of the three most important hospitals in Scotland and occupied a walled precinct measuring roughly 700m. As with the words 'street' and 'royal way' the 21st century visitor to Soutra must realise that the word 'hospital' had a rather different meaning during the Middle Ages. Although it was certainly a place offering medical care, it was also a hostel offering food and shelter for travellers. In addition, alms would have been dispensed there for the area's indigent population. According to contemporary charters Soutra was established by the Augustinians at the request of King Malcolm IV and was administered by the order with funding coming from their extensive estates - frequently augmented by benefactors who were grateful for the treatment they had received at the hands of the monks. Having said that, a contrary voice is raised by Dr Brian Moffat in the 1989 volume of SHARP. He states quite clearly that none..."of the published legal documentation from British Augustinian houses shows any link with Soutra." Much of the documentation from all monastic orders was destroyed during the Reformation so, sadly, clarity on this issue will remain elusive.

Who were the Augustinians?

St Augustine (354 - 430 AD) was born in Tagaste, now Souk-Ahras in modern day Algeria. After his conversion and baptism in 385 AD he lived a communal life with a group of fellow converts on his estate at Tagaste. Upon ordination he moved to Hippo and began to establish a monastic lifestyle which he further developed after he was consecrated bishop. He required the clergy in his Episcopal household to renounce private property and live a community life. His sister also entered a religious community and it was for his sister that he drew up his treatise on the virtues of chastity, concord and works of charity. This treatise became the Rule of St Augustine and underpinned all later Augustinian foundations in Europe. In England the famous holy shrine at Walsingham was an Augustinian foundation. Moving north there were many others - Cartmel, Conishead, Lanercost, Carlise, Iona, Saddell and Holywood to name a small selection - all followed the rule of St Augustine. For practical purposes the differences between an Augustinian house and, say, a Benedictine house at that time would have been hard to define. There was the same full liturgical round of choral offices but in many Augustinian houses the office used was that of the secular clergy which was shorter than the monastic office.

The diet was rather more generous than the Rule of St Benedict allowed and study, intellectual pursuits and research into, for example, medical treatments, were commended as acts of charity. Manual labour, both building work and agricultural work were also commended. At root the vocation of the Augustinians was the same as any other religious orders: to serve the spiritual needs of the community by prayer and service.

What was the religious historical background to the Soutra Foundation?

In the kingdom of the Scots, from roughly 900 to 1070 AD, the church was largely isolated from papal influence and the zeal of European reformers. Early forms of monasticism lingered on in the clergy communities of Culdees, (the servants of God), at places such as Iona and Scone. By no means could these be said to be monks - they took no monastic vows, were free to marry and own property.

The revival of monasticism in Scotland came about in the 100 years following the marriage in 1071 of King Malcolm III, (the prince perhaps better known for overthrowing the usurper Macbeth), to Margaret, the niece of Edward the Confessor. Margaret was later canonised for her support of the church and its monastic foundations. The chief royal contribution to monastic development was that of David I, King of Scots from 1124 - 1153 and Margaret's sixth son. David rebuilt the Scottish diocesan system and left his kingdom with ten bishoprics.

St Andrews was the prime see of Scotland with a large cathedral high on the old 'King's Mount' built during the 12th century. With David's full support this became monastic when a group of Austin Canons, i.e. members of the Augustinian order, moved in. The order had spread rapidly from its first establishment in Scone in 1120. The golden age of expansion ran up until 1286 when the problems of the succession to the crown began to lead towards war and an increase in lawlessness in the border regions. In this century and a half the religious orders, but in particular the Augustinians, set new and high standards in alms giving and care of the sick in monastic infirmaries and leper houses. Scottish monastic history from 1286 to the middle of the 16th century is too complex for a succinct summary and is sadly too short of historical record for absolute comments to be made.

The chief salient feature was intermittent but fierce war with England which seriously damaged foundations such as Soutra lying in vulnerable regions on main thoroughfares. What was an advantage in peace time became a disadvantage in times of war. The range of destruction and of warfare may be gauged when one considers that even so far south as the Furness peninsula the Cistercian Abbey of St Mary was sacked by the Scots.

The story of England's Reformation with its larger than life figures of King Henry VIII and Cromwell and the steady dissolution of monastic houses has no counterpart in Scotland. In Scotland the monasteries simply faded away as the reformers' idea that emphasis should be placed on an individual's relationship with God without the intermediary figure of a priest gradually took precedence. The doctrines of the reformers were inimical to monasticism: the real or alleged misconduct of monks and priests, was subject to mounting denunciation. Across Scotland there appeared to be evidence that the average community of brothers had lost the will to live up to its original vows and the behavioural standards of its first brethren. The heads of houses were more and more often laymen appointed as 'commendators' managing and profiting from monastic revenues.

By 1570 the authority of the Pope was abolished and the Mass along with it. The Protestant and Presbyterian Kirk was emerging. Dissolution had never been preached nor legislated for nor even officially sanctioned, rather, the communities steadily died out until, like Soutra, their buildings were used as a quarry for later local building work.

How did this affect Soutra?

Mention of the House of the Holy Trinity at Soutra in extant historical documents is fairly thin on the ground, The Vatican archives contain many supplications to Rome from the Scottish church: from these, particularly October 7th 1444, we can learn that the founders' intention was to establish a "...hospital for the reception of the poor.." The site was described as being in a remote place "...at the top of a hill.." Where there were often"...fierce winds and frequent cold spells..." The choice of location may reflect medieval society's suspicious fear of disease and pestilence

Documents of the time mention one Thomas Lauder (later Bishop of Dunkeld), as master of the Hospital of Soutra at the time of this supplication. He is on record as having made one of the first grant - of 5 shillings, towards the foundation of the Collegiate Church of the Holy Trinity in Edinburgh in 1462. In 1460 the Master of the Hospital had a more infamous character. His name was Stephen Fleming and he was so low in his character and behaviour that one of the Soutra brethren, by name Gilbert de Schechell, pleaded for him to be deposed. In his plea Gilbert de Schechell explained that Stephen Fleming had set aside his fear of God and his clerical modesty. He had rashly laid hands on a layman, (attacked him) some clerks also and even some priests, causing blood to flow. From this accusation, and other accusations recorded, we may deduce that the Master was both sexually incontinent and rather aggressive. In response to this accusation the Scottish crown seized Soutra's estates thus depriving it of its means of income. These same estates were later given to Trinity College Hospital in Edinburgh providing early support for the beginning of Edinburgh's development into a centre for medical research. A nice continuity. The House of the Holy Trinity sank slowly into poverty and dereliction functioning as a local centre for alms giving until about 1650.

In 1686 the Pringle family of Soutra/Beatman's Acre decided to use part of the precinct as a family burial vault. It is important to be aware that the building seen at Soutra today is not the remnant of any part of the medieval church or hospital. It is a burial vault known in Scotland as an 'aisle' and was built using a small amount of masonry from the crumbled monastic buildings plus local rubble. These aisles became popular in 17th century Scotland when family burials inside churches were no longer allowed.

As we have previously noted, Soutra's high moorland position would have made it a bleak place during the winter months. The Augustinian order founded a hospital for pilgrims in the 11th century upon the Great St. Bernard's pass. Local historians have dubbed Soutra the 'St Bernard's' of Scotland. Within the precinct there was one healing well known as Trinity Well and there was a second one known as 'Prior's Well' but a short way away from the church. Trinity Well was thought to have waters of a miraculous nature: James Hunter in his work 'Fala and Soutra', including a history of the Domus de Soltre' says that the spring there was a "...popular resort..." for local people and pilgrims from which the brethren acquired "...some fame..."

In SHARP 1989 (The Third Report on Researches into the Medieval Hospital at Soutra p14) we read that these two wells are mentioned many times in the 60 Soutra charters. No other source of water is named for the foundation so we must surmise that the well, along with collected rainwater, met the needs of the population. If we consider that large groups of travellers -

including armies with their baggage trains - were accommodated at Soutra there was quite clearly a large and dependable source of water. We know from the same charters that Soutra owned, ran and rented both a water mill and a windmill. The watermill is in ruins on the Linn Dean Burn 2.5kms to the north. The Soutra summit stands on an exposed escarpment endowed with the unlimited wind power ideal for windmills. Again, from these charters we learn there was a pomerium (orchard) and a vinea (vineyard). In addition to apples and grapes the inhabitants of Soutra had access to a more varied range of plants for food and for medication than might have been expected.

Over recent years Soutra has been the subject of extensive archaeological excavation by the team led by Dr Brian Moffat. Extensive examination of the hospital waste has revealed the use of many plants for medicine and for cooking that clearly have an overseas origin, cloves and nutmeg being but two examples. In SHARP 1998 Dr Moffat quotes from Soutra Charter No. 11 and explains that in return for the use of a piece of land near Threeburnfold - lying between Lauderdale and Gala water - the brethren of Soutra undertook to pay the Abbot and Convent of Dryburgh Abbey one pound of cumin and one pound of pepper a St James's Fair, Roxburgh each year. It should be understood that spices at this time were a form of currency with rents in Europe being often commuted into their spice equivalent.

On page 24 of the above volume Dr Moffat explains that he and his team have searched the extant records of Augustinian houses especially in northern Britain, to see which spices were being bought and used. In one of these, Bolton Priory, W. Yorkshire we learn that cinnamon and ginger were being used. By means of this kind of research it is hoped to gain an insight into what may also have been in use at Soutra. In the enclosure around Soutra Aisle many native and non-native species of plant have been found growing. An insight into these herbs is no part of the remit of the present chapter and will be dealt with in depth elsewhere. Suffice to say that there is evidence of a combination of henbane, hemlo and opium poppy seeds being used in a maceration producing an early form of anaesthetic drink probably used in cases of amputation or for dealing with great pain caused by other disease such as cancer.

Bibliography:

1. Annie Dunlop, Ian MacLauchian, David and Ian Cowan, Editors Calendar of Scottish Supplications to Rome 1433 - 1447 Vol. IV. University of Glasgow Press. 1983 pps: 266-7.

2. Brian Moffat, G. Euart and L. Euan. SHARP Practise Edinburgh, several volumes 1986-9

3. C. H. Lawrence. Medieval Monasticism. Longman 1989.

4. Lionel Butler and Chris Given. Wilson Medieval Monasteries of Great Britain Michael Joseph 1979.

More surprisingly is the discovery in the monastery hospital waste of a combination of ergot and juniper berries in a stone culvert which have been interpreted as a parturient preparation. (Aid to child birth).

Finally, the personnel at Soutra can only be surmised from what is known of other Augustinian foundations. We know there was a master and beneath him there would have been the customary hierarchy of monastic officers. The special task to which each official was assigned was called an 'obedience' and he himself was called an 'obedientiary'.

The number of these depended on the size of the foundation but we can reasonably assume at Soutra that certain key officers would have been necessary for the running of the establishment. First in importance was the sacrist who looked after the fabric of the church and oversaw repairs and refurbishments to the structure and the contents. The almoner would have to have been a person of significance at Soutra as he dispensed alms and other forms of relief to the poor. The cellarer's responsibility was to oversee the supply of food, drink and fuel to all parts of the community. The guest master had the responsibility of providing accommodation for the continual stream of visitors which could vary from prelates to paupers. At Soutra the infirmarian and his sub-infirmarians would have held a special position. He had charge of what was, in effect, a parallel establishment mostly situated to the east of the main complex and having its own dormitory and chapel. These buildings housed the sick, the elderly, those who had been bled for the sake of their health, (there is evidence of blood discovered in the hospital waste) and those too infirm to take part in the work of the monastery. An indeterminate number of lay brothers would have also been there to provide the supporting roles of labourers and auxiliary helpers in all areas where the need arose.

Conclusion

Thus far we have considered Soutra within its broader geographical, historical and cultural background.

Let us move onto a more detailed examination of the kind of herbal/medicinal practices which took place at the hospital at Soutra.

A medieval monastery's approach to running an infirmary

The Hospital in History, 'Medieval English Hospitals' by Martha Carlin provides an overview of 1,103 Medieval Hospitals.

They fall into four categories:

1. Leper hospitals
2. Almshouses
3. Respite for poor travellers and pilgrims
4. For the care of the non-leprous sick poor

Only limited medical care was available but generally patients were provided with bed rest, warmth, cleanliness and an adequate diet.

'Development and Change in English Hospitals 1100-1500 AD' by Miri Rubin indicates that the question of medical practices in medieval hospitals is a difficult and puzzling one as one can read the greater part of a full hospital archive covering hundreds of years and yet encounter not one mention of drugs purchased or payments to physicians or surgeons. Although it is understood tha many of the medicines used at this time would have been grown i herb gardens within the monastery or bought in for culinary uses as well as medicinal purposes.

This lack of information about medicine and surgery used during this time in monasteries makes the excavations at Soutra all the more valuable.

Some useful information has been discovered in 'Plant Names of Medieval England' and 'Popular Medicine in C13 England' both by Tony Hunt, this last publication giving over 1,000 recipes and medical prescriptions.

Another important reference book available at this time was Macer Floridus, written in verse, a useful handbook for any physician. It lists 105 herbs and spices and their uses, there is som variation in the order and content of the other Macer books still i existence and although its origins are somewhat obscure - some even attribute it to Pliny the Elder. Macer Floridus is hardly original in the description of plants and their medicinal propertie Dioscorides also did this in his series of books - De Materia Medica. In fact approximately 2,000 verses of De Materia Medica can be directly attributed to the Historia Naturalis 77 AD by Pliny The author behind the collection of verses known as Macer is probably Odo of Meung who may have lived in the first half of th

C11. Manitis suggests that the traces of Greek used in Macer prove that he - the author - had possibly been to school at Orleans or Fleury, both of which are quite near Meung. The absence of any mention of Avicenna or of his herbal remedies or indeed any other Arab physician indicate that this book was written before the establishment of Arabic medicine in the west i.e. before the beginning of the C10. In addition,the famous teaching hospital in Salerno is not mentioned in Macer but there are a number of references to Macer in Regimen Sanitatis - a collection of writings from Salerno. The significance of Macer is due to various references within the book which show it must have been originally written towards the end of the C9, the book was much copied and many monastic houses list numerous copies within their libraries making it one of the most widely available medical books at this time. There are still 57 manuscript copies or partial copies recorded, the oldest is in Vienna possibly written around 1150.

The first printed edition is dated 1477 and was produced in Naples, many of these printed versions contained woodcut images of the herbs and on the title page a woodcut of a writing monk surrounded by books and a flask. Two of the early printed versions have some beautiful engravings of the herbs and are to be found in the British Library. The majority are in Germany. Some are more decorative and others much simpler, often the scribe will comment on the value of a certain remedy if he/she has found it particularly useful and distance themselves from herbs that they probably hadn't used and that are potentially dangerous - black and white hellebore fall into this category.

A number of medieval scientific authors mention the poem in their works, it was possibly one of the reference books that Hildegard von Bingen used for the section 'De Plantis' in her work 'Physica'.

Throughout Macer there are many comments referencing great physicians and authorities who back up the authors opinions on the uses of various herbs.

The following names appear in the text but not in history (as we know it). It is to be supposed that they are corruptions of other names or, possibly, inventions by the author.

Caton; Mellicus; Putagoras; Menemacus; Crisppus; Amasilans;

Strabus; Sexus Niger; Prosius; Vribasius;

There are a few referenced authorities who have survived through the ages :

Mithridates

Mithridates VI was the king of Pontius in Asia Minor 120BC-63BC He was also known as Mithridates the Great on account of his victories against the great Roman generals Sulla, Pompey the Great and Lucullus. He is also famous for his decision to guard against death by poisoning by taking increasing sub-lethal doses of poison until he could tollerate lethal doses. These experiments later led to an antidote which could be universally applied known as the 'Antidotum Mthridaticum', this antidote was used in medicine for the next 1900 years and was known as 'theriaca'. The Merriam-Webster medical dictionary defines therica as an antidote to poison containing about 70 ingredients pulverised and added to honey to be used as an electuary. It was also known as Venice treacle.

Ironically when Mithridates finally suffered defeat at the hands of Pompey and wished to kill himself he was unable to do so owing to his immunity to poisons. He was obliged to request that one of his servants stab him with a sword.

Xenocrates

Xenocrates was a Greek physician of Aphrodisias in Glicia who lived around the middle of the C1. He wrote several pharmaceutica treatises and was on several occasions quoted by Galen who decried his use of unpleasant ingredients such as human brains and excrement, in his remedies.

Asclepius / Asklepios / Aesculapius

Asclepius was the ancient Greek god of medicine and the son of the sun god Apollo. It is thought that this divinity was originally based on a famous healer whose origins are obscure but who was held, during his lifetime, to be more a god than a man and was credited with being able to raise the dead. Many temples were built and dedicated to Asclepius.

The two translations that I have seen, and spent the greater part of my time studying are: Gosta Frisk, 'translation into Middle English' and Bruce Pepper Flood's Ph.D. in which dissertation the English translation of Macer's work focuses on some of the manuscripts and printed versions of the book Macer Floridus which are still in existence. Macer Floridus de Viribus Herbarium was translated by Ludwig Choulant in 1832, this translation has some additional herbs included at the end of the book which he says are written in a different hand and obviously added at a later date by a previous owner of the book. These additions are also found in editions of Macer translated by Conaris and Ranzowius which place the probable date of these extra herbal inclusions at some time in the C15.

These additional herbs and other elements are:- Araron/*Colubrina*, Agrimony/*Agrimonia europea*, Elder/*Sambucus nigra*, Water lily/*Nymphaea*, Bean/*Fabia*, Filbert nut/*Avellana*, Blackberry/*Batus sive rubus*, Myrica/*Tamarisc*, White Willow/*Salix alb*a, Fumatory/*fumaria*, Excrement/*Fimus*, Cheese/*Caseus*, Spiders web/*Aracneae tela*, Snails/ *Cochleae*, Stags horn/*Cornu cervi*, Sulphur/*Sulphur vivum*, Alum/*Alumen*

Some of these herbs fill glaring omissions in the original Macer and others have gone out of use over the years, but the inclusion of alum and sulphur nod towards Paracelsus (considered to be the father of chemical medicine) and his enthusiasm for using small amounts of minerals in his medicines.

The layout and information in Macer is very similar in both Frisk's and Flood's works, indicating that the original 77 chapters or verses have remained consistent throughout the centuries. The purpose of both projects seem to have been focussed more on the language and the origins of Macer's book rather than looking at the herbal remedies in any detail.

There are some herbs mentioned that are difficult to identify with certainty and others which have been left out although their remains have been found in the medical waste in the drain at Soutra. The absence of St. John's Wort is striking as it appears several times in Soutra's drains combined with valerian - a herb that only merited a brief comment in Macer - a mixture that is used today to treat anxiety and depression. So, Macer is not a complete herbal as far as Scottish herbs are concerned. This is another indication that the herbal information found in this book was derived from sources which were based on herbs found growing in a warmer climate. Which explains some of the 'gaps' in the selection of herbs found in Macer - where is hawthorn, or dandelion?

Macer is certainly not as detailed as Dioscorides' work which is extensive and runs to many volumes making it more of a reference work than a useful handbook - which seems to have been the role that Macer's book occupied. It is interesting to note the common conditions that were treated in the Middle Ages and to compare these with the ailments we see today, obviously Holy Fire has faded into history although the last outbreak in Europe was in France in the 1950s, and ergot poisoning still occurs occasionally in Africa if there has been a particularly wet harvest.

The opportunity to comment that a particular treatment will 'kill or cure' has also gone out of fashion. But in times when information was harder to access it was important to know the safety or otherwise of the herbs you were using.

The herbs mentioned in Macer have been carefully checked and identified using all available information, but there may be inaccuracies with herbal identification.

Macer floridus

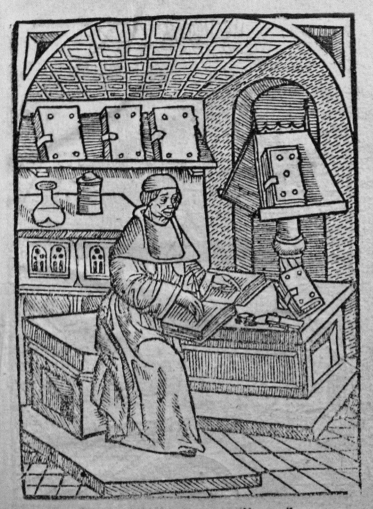

De viribus herbar

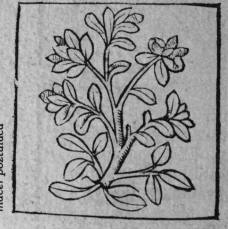

macer poztulaca

21st Century
Modern Macer
Translation

Page 4:
Essential herbs
numbers 1-66

Page 121:
Spices
numbers 67-78

Page 138:
Not to be forgotten herbs
numbers 79-105

Contents of Macer herbs

Herb number. *Latin name* | Medieval name | **Common name**

Essential herbs

1. *Artemisia vulgaris* | **Mugwort**
2. *Artemisia abrotanum* | **Southernwood**
3. *Artemisia absinth* | **Wormwood**
4. *Urtica dioica* | **Nettle**
5. *Allium sativum* | Garlik | **Garlic**
6. *Plantago major* | *Plantago lanceolata* | Planteyn | **Plantain** | **Ribwort**
7. *Ruta graviolens* | Rewe | **Rue**
8. *Aristolochia clematis* | Smerewort | **Clematis**
9. *Apium graviolens* | Smalache | **Celery**
10. *Juniperus communis* | Saueyne | **Juniper**
11. *Allium ampeloprasum* | Leeke | **Leek**
12. *Nepeta cataria* | Nepis | **Catmint**
13. *Foeniculum vulgare* | **Fennel**
14. *Lactuca virosa* | **Lettuce**
15. *Rosa canina* | **Rose**
16. *Lilium album* | **Lily**
17. *Satureja hortensis* | Sanuerye | **Savory**
18. *Inula helenium* | Horsehelene | **Elecampane**
19. *Salvia officinalis* | **Sage**
20. *Hyssopus officinalis* | Isope | **Hyssop**
21. *Iris germanica* | Gladene | **Iris**
22. *Althea rosea* | Vyldmalwe | **Hollyhock**
23. *Pimpinella anisum* | Anyse | **Aniseed**
24. *Stachys betonica* | Betoyne | **Wood Betony**
25. *Brassica* | Coul | **Cabbage**
26. *Allium cepa* | Oynones | **Onions**
27. *Brassica nigra* | *Sinapsis alba* | Senueye | **Mustard**
28. *Piper album* | **White Pepper**
29. *Nasturtium officianale* | Nasturtium | **Watercress**
30. *Viola odorata* | **Violet**
31. *Papaver somniferens* | **Poppy**
32. *Coriandrum sativum* | Coriundre | **Coriander**
33. *Atriplex patula* | Arage | Arach | **Lesser Wild Arach**
34. *Mentha piperita* | Mynte | **Mint**
35. *Pastinacea sativa* | **Skyrwhit**
36. *Anthriscus cerefolium* | Cerfoile | **Chervil**
37. *Rumex patiens* | Dokke | **Dock**
38. *Nigella sativa* | Kockul | **Nigella**
39. *Conium maculatum* | **Hemlock**
40. *Mentha pulegium* | Pyloile | Brother Wort | **Pennyroyal**
41. *Thymus vulgaris* | Persile | **Thyme**
42. *Centaurium erythraea* | Centory | **Centaury**
43. *Teucrium chamaedrys* | Gamodreos | **Germander**
44. *Dracunculus vulgaris* | Dragance | **Dragonwort**
45. *Matricaria recutita* | Chamomille | **Chamomile**
46. *Gonecera periclinenum* | *Levisticum officinali* | Wodebynd | **Lovage**
47. *Rumex acetosa* | Sorell | **Sorrel**
48. *Rumex acetosella* | Iubarbe | **Sheep Sorrel**
49. *Portulaca oleracea* | **Purslane**
50. *Saponaria officianalis* | Bysshopswort | **Soapwort**
51. *Anchusa italica* | *Anchusa atrigosa* | Langedboef | **Italian Bugloss**
52. *Puliole haunt* | **Oregano**

Not to be fogotten herbs

53. *Marubium vulgare* | Horhoune | **Horehound**
54. *Asarum europeum* | Softe | **European Ginger**
55. *Cyperus articulatus* | Cyperus | **Sweet Cyprus**
56. *Paeonia officinale* | Pyoney | **Peony**
57. *Melissa officialis* | Balm | **Lemon Balm**
58. *Senecio vulgaris* | Groundswely | **Groundsel**
59. *Cheledonium majus* | *Ranunculus ficaria* | Celydone | **Greater & Lesser Celandine**
60. *Isatis tictora* | Gwade | **Wode**
61. *Helleborus alba* | White Ellebore | **White Hellebore**
62. *Helleborus niger* | Black Ellebore | **Black Hellebore**
63. *Verbena officinalis* | Verveyn | **Vervane**
64. *Solanum nigrum* | Morell | **Black Nightshade**
65. *Hyoscyamus niger* | **Henbane**
66. *Althea officianalis* | Hocke | Althea | **Marshmallow**

Spices

67. *Piper nigrum* | **Pepper**
68. *Parietaria officinalis* | Peletre | **Pellitory of The Wall**
69. *Zingiber officinale* | Gyngyrere | **Ginger**
70. *Cuminium cyminum* | Comyn | **Cumin**
71. *Alpinia officianale* | **Galingale**
72. *Curcuma longa* | Zeduale | **Turmeric**
73. *Syzygium aromaticum* | Clowe gelofre | **Clove**
74. *Cinnamomum verum* | Canel | **Cinnamon**
75. *Costus arabicus* | Coste | **Of the Ginger family**
76. *Nardostachys jatamans* | **Spikenard**
77. *Boswellia sacra* | Frankensence | **Frankincense**
78. *Aloe vulgaris* | **Aloe**

79. *Sanicula europa* | **Sanicle**
80. *Pimpernella saxifrage* | Pympernolle | **Pimpernel**
81. *Gentian amarelle* | Baldmoyne | **Gentian**
82. *Beta vulgaris* | Beta | **Beet**
83. *Calendula officinalis* | Rhodewort | **Marigold**
84. *Tanacetum vulgaris* | **Tansy**
85. *Laurus noblis* | Laureole | **Laurel**
86. *Glycyrrhiza glabra* | **Liquorice**
87. *Myristica fragrans* | Notemuge | **Nutmeg**
88. *Myrtus communis* | Mirtus | **Myrtle**
89. *Crocus sativum* | Safron | **Saffron**
90. *Carum carvi* | **Caraway**
91. *Pimpinella saxifraga* | Saxifrage | **Lesser Burnet**
92. *Geum urbanum* | **Bennet**
93. *Oreganum dictamnus* | Ditayne | **Dittany**
94. *Tanacetum parthenium* | Featherfoy | **Feverfew**
95. *Mentha longifolia* | Bawme | **Horsemint**
96. *Scrophularia nodosa* | Mille-Morbia | **Figwort**
97. *Brionia dioica* | Nepe | **Bryony**
98. *Raphanus sativus* | Raddish | **Radish**
99. *Trigonella foenumgraecum* | **Fenugreek**
100. *Salvia sclarea* | Sclareye | **Clary Sage**
101. *Nigella sativav* | **Git**
102. *Asarum europeum* | **Azara**
103. *Valeriana officinalis* | **Valerian**
104. *Lupinus alba* | Lupinus | **Lupin**
105. *Datura stramonium* | **Thorn Apple**

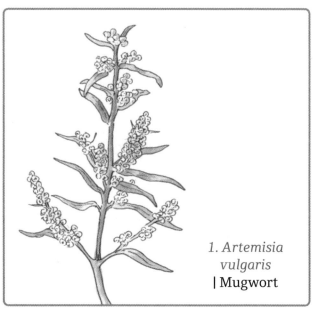

1. Artemisia vulgaris
| Mugwort

1.
Artemisia vulgaris
| **Mugwort**

Mugwort is known as artesmisia after Diana also known as Artemis.

PRIMARILY

This herb is especially useful for women's illnesses.

Taken as a decoction it can bring on a woman's periods, whether it is drunk as the fresh herb ground up and mixed with wine or the green herb is bruised and wrapped over her womb over night.

It can bring on a miscarriage either when it is drunk or when applied as a poultice.

It softens the hardness of the womb and helps reduce tumours.

As a drink it also increases urination and dissolves kidney stones.

It helps heal liver conditions including jaundice if it is drunk frequently.

Pliny praises this herb when mixed with wine for helping recovery from excessive use of opium.

It is said that drinking an infusion of this herb will protect you from poisons and that the protection extends to preventing wild beasts from seizing and biting you.

When its root is hung from your neck you will be protected from poisonous toads and frogs.

When ground up and mixed with wine this herb will comfort the stomach and act as a tonic to all the inner organs of the body.

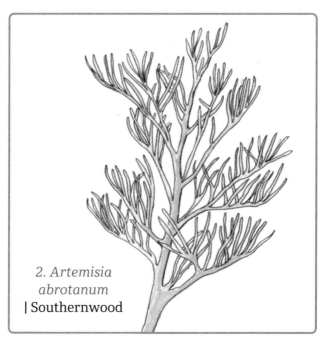

2. Artemisia abrotanum | Southernwood

2.
Artemisia abrotanum | **Southern-wood**

Southernwood is also known as artesmisia after Diana also known as Artemis.

Its smell causes serpents to flee and provides protection from their poisons.

PRIMARILY

This herb is helpful for treating lung conditions, a boiled decoction of this herb when drunk helps those who have difficulty breathing and it helps ease coughs.

It is also helpful for ailments of the womb when the fresh herb is infused in wine and drunk.

It also heals sciatica and brings on a woman's periods.

When taken at the onset of a child's fever it will have a cooling effect.

By drinking this infusion frequently you will kill the worms of the stomach.

Boiling quinces and bread together with southernwood will ease the pain of the eyes when this is applied as a poultice.

Thorns and splinters can be removed easily if this mixture is applied to the area as it is or blended with fat.

Placed on a pillow this herb acts as a love charm.

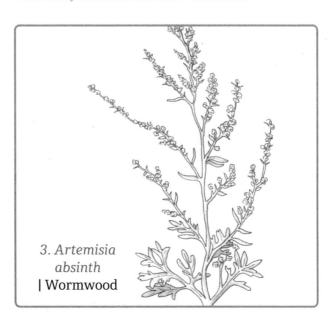

3. Artemisia absinth | Wormwood

3.
Artemisia absinth
| Wormwood

Hot in the first degree.
Again, this is named
with reference to Diana,
also known as Artemis.

PRIMARILY

For worms and a laxative ~
It destroys worms in the belly and makes a laxative and eases aches and pains of the womb.

Drink wormwood and it makes you piss.

For women's periods ~
Take spikenard and wormwood, grind them together, steep with wine, drink it and it will bring on a woman's period quickly.

Take wormwood or similar, add the seed of rue, salt and pepper and grind together, mix with wine, heat and drink ~ this will relieve discomforts of the stomach.

For the breast ~
Mix together wormwood and iris and drink and it helps the breast wonderfully.

Jaundice ~
Eat raw wormwood and celery together ~ this will heal jaundice.

For the poison of hemlock or of toadstool ~ eat or drink wormwood and it neutralises the poison of both these things.

Drink wormwood and it helps protect you against bites of venomous beasts.

Eyes ~
Mix wormwood with honey, apply to the eyes and it makes them clear and heals cloudiness/cataracts and the swellings of the eyes.

Ears ~

If you are going deaf, infuse wormwood in hot water and let the vapour go into the ear and this will have a healing effect. If the ears suppurate mix wormwood with honey and apply to the ear and it should heal.

Swollen throat ~

If cheeks are swollen bruise wormwood with honey and apply it to the swelling.

For wounds ~

Bruising the herb and applying it to fresh wounds will help them heal, it is also good for the head or fractures of the head, grind and infuse wormwood in wine and honey and make a plaster and apply it to the wounds of the head and it will heal them.

For breaks/fractures ~

Drink the juice of wormwood with an equal amount of wine and you will heal quickly.

For the sore groin ~

Lay on a linen cloth some wormwood and bind it about the legs and this will ease the severe ache of the groin.

To aid sleep ~

The smell of wormwood acts as a soporific and it is also effective if it is laid under the head.

To make women beautiful ~

The ash of wormwood will bleach the skin if it is mixed with oil, apply this ointment frequently to achieve a pale complexion.

Put wormwood in a chest and it will keep the moths away.

Tongue ~

Bruise wormwood with honey and put some under the tongue, it will heal the ache and the swelling of this area.

This same medicine will heal paleness and discolouring that appears about the outside of the eye.

For the spleen ~

A plaster of wormwood made with honey softens the hardness of the spleen.

Make a decoction of wormwood and drink it, this will dry up the skin that the child lies in within his mother's womb and enable the afterbirth to come away easily.

For the stomach ~

Infuse green wormwood in oil and massage into the stomach to ease discomfort.

This herb comforts and strengthens the stomach in whatever way it is taken.

The best way ~ soak it in rain water and drink it cold.

This will help various sicknesses of the stomach.

Let wormwood lie and soak in wine for a while and with this liquid dilute the ink and neither moths nor rats will gnaw the book that is written with this ink.

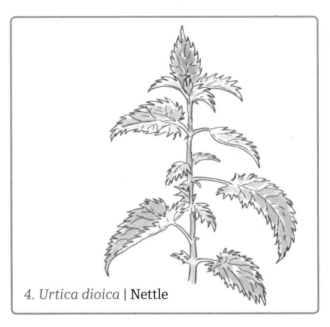

4. Urtica dioica | Nettle

4.

Urtica dioica | Nettle

The nettle in Greek is known as acaliphe. It is extremely hot and therefore it is known as vrtica in Latin, because it will burn the fingers that handle it.

PRIMARILY

For jaundice ~
Drink a nettle infusion to heal jaundice.

For colic pains ~
Eat and drink nettle seeds with honey to ease colic.

For coughs ~
Drink nettle seed tea frequently and it will heal chronic coughs.

For the lungs ~
It eases the cold of the lungs and the ache of the womb and various swellings. For all these pains use powdered nettle leaf or nettle seed mixed well with honey, it is also effective if the green herb is frequently drunk infused in wine.

For wounds and swellings/tumours ~
Bruise nettle leaves and blend with salt to make a plaster, this will cleanse infected wounds and soothe swellings.

For dog bites and cancer ~
This plaster is effective in healing dog bites and cancers and the illness called parotid (swelling of the parotid glands in the neck) also dislocations and this plaster also repairs and heals flesh that has been torn from the bone.

For humours ~
And this dries up 'noxious humours.'

For gout and limbs ~
Bruised nettle root infused in wine reduces swelling of the spleen and is an excellent treatment for gout, it is good for all the sicknesses of the toes; if it is made into a plaster or infused in oil, massage the limbs and toes with the ointment .

For a nose bleed ~
So great is the heat in nettles that if you rub the outside of someone's nose that is bleeding with the juice of a nettle, it will stop the bleeding.

Put the juice of the nettle leaf into the nose, and it will cause a nose bleed.

Make a drink of nettles and myrrh and it will bring on a women's period.

Mix nettles or nettle seeds with wine and it will provoke lechery, it will have a stronger effect if you mix it with salt, honey and pepper and drink all this mixed together in wine.

The four footed beast that will not stand for her mate should be rubbed with nettles, and soon it will stand still to the male. This is how stimulating the natural heat of nettles can be. Rub well a barren beasts cervix with nettle leaves or with the juice of it and the beast will conceive.

Nettle seed should be gathered in August and dried and then you will have an excellent medicine available throughout the year.

For pleurisy ~
Make a drink of nettle seeds mixed with honey, and this will heal the sickness that is known as pleurisy.

For breast and lungs ~
This mixture is also very beneficial to the breast and lungs. Drink with wine, and it will increase urination.

For a laxative ~
Infuse nettles in oil and drink the infusion and it will ease constipation.

For the mouth ~
Take nettle seeds and roll them in the mouth and this will reduce the swellings of that part of the mouth that is known as the uvula.

To encourage sweating ~
Massage with an oil that has had nettles infused in it, this will bring on sweating.

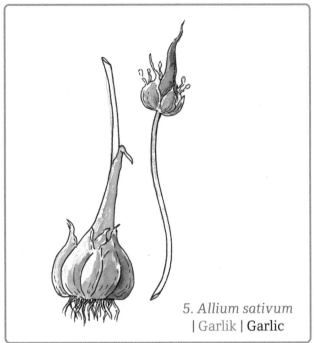

5. *Allium sativum*
| Garlik | Garlic

5.
Allium sativum
| Garlik
| Garlic

Garlic is hot and dry in the fourth degree

PRIMARILY

For dog bites ~
Blend garlic with honey and it will heal dog bites and also snake and adder bites.

Eat garlic or apply it to a sore place, and it will heal all bites.

For worms ~
The odour of crushed garlic drives away harmful worms, boil garlic in wine and put into it a little vinegar and drink it; this will kill worms in the womb and the stomach/intestines.

For cold that has 'burst out' ~ with the same mixture you can heal someone who is very cold.

For venomous beast bites ~
Warm garlic cloves in oil, and this oil will heal the bites of deadly and venomous beasts if the area of the bite is rubbed with the oil.

For the bladder ~
Rub the pubic region with garlic soaked in mulsa/wine and vinegar and this will heal any swelling or discomfort of the bladder.

Another use for this poultice ~
Crushed garlic warmed in water and applied as a plaster to the penis (pubic region) will heal infection or inflammation. Crushed garlic infused in a bath will help a woman after giving birth to a child, to release the afterbirth. In a similar way inhaling the fumes from heated garlic will have a similar effect.

For diseased lungs ~
Infuse garlic cloves in goat's milk and eat the cloves and drink the milk ~ this will heal many lung conditions. Also eating the garlic raw will be equally effective.

For dropsy/heart failure ~
Heat garlic with centaury and it will help support anyone with heart failure by drying up 'watery humours' (fluid retention.)

For nephritis and kidney stones ~
Warm garlic with coriander and wine, eat and drink this to treat nephritis, kidney stones and also for kidney infections.

For jaundice ~
This is good for the kidneys or for jaundice and it makes the womb and stomach 'soft'.

For headaches ~
Infuse garlic with beans, grind the mixture up and make a plaster of the mixture, apply it to the head or the temples and it will ease headaches.

Eat garlic first thing in the morning with wine and throughout the day you will have no need to fear coming to harm from any form of water.

For the ear ~
Blend garlic with goose grease and melt it and when it is warm put it in the ear and it will ease earache and is guaranteed to also improve hearing.

For coughs ~
Infuse garlic in water and eat this frequently and it will ease coughs and shortness of breath.

For the bowel ~
Garlic and mercury, blend them together and eat the mixture; this will heal the sickness that is called tensamon.

For boils ~
Grind garlic with pig fat and make a plaster of the mixture and it will ease boils and swellings if you frequently apply this mixture to the area.

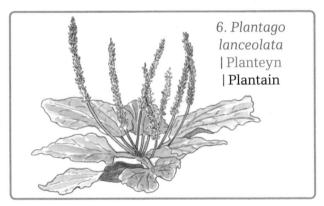

6. *Plantago major* | Planteyn | Plantain

6. *Plantago lanceolata* | Planteyn | Plantain

6.

Plantago major | Plantago lanceolata | Planteyn | Plantain | Ribwort

Plantain is cold and dry in the third degree.

PRIMARILY

For wounds ~
Greater plantain will dry moist wounds and cleanse infected wounds if it is mixed with honey and salt and soaked in vinegar and applied to the wound.

For flux/dysentery ~
Take this herb and another and prepare them in the same way and eat them and it will staunch haemorrhages from the womb and the flux of the womb that aches. It has the same effect if it is applied externally as a plaster or poultice.

For black spots ~
Rub any black spot with plantain juice and it will return it to its original colour.

For burns ~
Blend plantain juice with sheep's milk and it will heal burns and scalds.

For dog bites ~
Use bruised plantain leaves to heal dog bites and soothe swellings.

For kernel ~
Bruise this herb with salt and it will heal deep ulcers if it is applied to the area.

For the dropsy ~
Cook plantain and eat it, it is helpful in easing the effects of heart failure and helps heal anyone who has a 'chincough' or epilepsy.

For wounds in the mouth ~
Hold the juice of plantain in the mouth for a long time and roll it around well; it cleanses foul /infected wounds in the mouth.

For fistulas ~
Hold the juice of plantain in the fistula, and it will heal it. The juice of plantain is good for earache if it is held in the ear for a while.

For Holy Fire/ergot poisoning ~
With the juice of plantain wash the place which is affected by the ailment that is known as Holy Fire, and it will soothe and heal it.

For coughs ~
Drink the juice of plantain frequently, and it will heal coughs and ease conditions that cause 'blood spitting'.

For the bloody dysentery ~
Take the juice of plantain by enema, and it will heal dysentery.

For eyes ~
Anoint the eyes frequently with plantain juice and this will ease swellings and is cooling for the eyes

For the gums ~
Chew greater plantain leaves and this will heal bleeding gums. And in the same way it eases toothache.

For headaches ~
Hang the root of this herb about the neck and it will ease headaches. Soak wool in the warm juice of plantain and place it on a woman's cervix to stop her haemorrhaging blood or any other discharge.

For scorpions stings ~
Grind up and apply plantain root to the area that a scorpion has stung and it will heal it. To all the previously mentioned illnesses a decoction of this herb will heal them. But even better is the seed of it soaked in wine.

For the bladder ~
Drink this plantain juice and it will heal the ache of the bladder and the kidneys.

For coughs ~
It is said that if you carry the root of plantain around your neck you will never suffer from a cough - as long as you are wearing the root.

For tertian fever ~
Take three roots of this herb and grind them up, mix them with three cups of wine and with the same amount of water, give this to anyone that has fever before the quaking develops and in this way tertian fever can be cured.

Here note that this cup is known in Latin as ciatus, and ciatus holds as much as half a hen egg shell can hold.

Plantain lanceolata is good for easing the swellings of the nostril, if you apply the juice of this herb or make a plaster of it.

For swellings of the eye ~
In the same way it is good for easing the swellings of the eyes, if it is applied every day for nine days with soft wool.

For ache of the womb ~
Lay upon the womb the warm juice of this herb and wash the area with it.

For worms of the womb ~
Drink frequently the juice of this herb by itself or mix it with old pig fat and apply it to the area in the form of a poultice.

For swellings, for parotid and for wounds ~
It is effective in easing swellings that are hard and it reduces swellings of the parotid glands (salivary glands) and heals fresh and new wounds.

For fevers ~
Drink the juice of this herb two hours before the attack and it will heal the ague/fever. Drink the juice of this herb and it will help release the afterbirth.

For aching feet ~
Grind this herb with wine or vinegar and make a plaster of it and cover the aching foot with it to ease the ache. The seed of this herb will have a similar effect if it is drunk and also the juice if it is mixed with raisons.

For the bladder ~
This herb is good for various sicknesses of the bladder due to its drying effect.

For swellings ~
For swellings and dislocations anywhere within the body.

Greater Plantain is known in Greek as *arnoglossa*. It has leaves like a lambs tongue. There are two types of plantain; the first is known as the more/greater and the other is known as the lesser. And this lesser is known as lanceolata because the leaves are shaped like a spear.

It is said *arnoglossa* has the greater might and virtue.

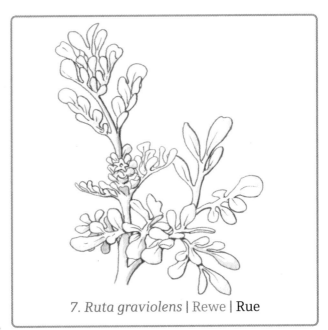

7. *Ruta graviolens* | Rewe | **Rue**

7.

Ruta graviolens | Rewe | **Rue**

Hot and dry to the third degree.

Good for the stomach.

PRIMARILY

For the Guts ~

Blend rue in a little butter and oil and it will ease the swelling of the womb if it is applied warm. In the same way it will heal diseases of the colon and all illnesses that are within the body.

If you infuse green rue in oil and when warm apply this to the mouth of the vagina it will heal any swelling present. Hold it in with an enema and this will heal the swellings of the bowels, rue is most effective if drunk with wine.

Birth ~

Rue will speed the delivery of the child and suppresses lechery if it is drunk, also it brings on a woman's periods: soak rue in water and the fourth part vinegar and drink this mixture. It will ease pain in the belly.

Seethe/infuse rue in oil and eat it or drink it and this will destroy the worms in the womb.

Lungs ~

It helps the lungs and the breast and also the ache and disease of the ribs known as pleurisy.

Arthritis/gout ~

It will ease the gout that is known as arthritis. And also fevers, if you make a tea of it and drink it.

Dropsy/heart failure ~

Soak long figs and rue in wine and the resulting liquor is good
for anyone that has dropsy/heart failure.

For eyes ~

Eaten raw it will clarify the sight. But it is more effective if you
make an ointment of the juice of rue and the juice of fennel with
the bile of a cockerel mixed with honey - the equivalent amount
to that of the rue, and with this mixture anoint the eyes
frequently. (A similar mixture taken from a Saxon herbal The
Leech Book of Bald has shown signs of being as effective as
antibiotics in treating Staphylococcal infections of the eye)

Head aches ~

Blend the juice of rue with the oil of roses and ewe fat and this
ointment will ease headaches if it is applied to the head.

Nose ~

Squeeze out the juice of rue and hold it in at the nostrils during
a nose bleed and it will stop the bleeding.

And it will also ease the scabs that are called herpes and the
swellings that rise out of the nostrils.

Earache ~

Warm the juice of rue and the rind/husk of a pomegranate and
hold it in to the ear and it will heal earache.

Holy Fire/Ergot poisoning ~

Mix the juice of rue with oil, vinegar and ewe fat and myrrh and
this confection if it is used repeatedly will heal the condition
known as Holy Fire.

Head injuries ~

This ointment will heal fractures to the head out of which runs a
fatty humour/liquid.

For the bollocks/testicles ~

Grind rue with bay leaves and make a plaster and this will ease
swellings of the testicles.

For all the parts of the body ~

Take pepper, cumin and nitrum in equal weight and of rue as
much as of all these three together but make sure that the cumin
is well soaked in sharp vinegar and that all of these are left to
dry on a hot plate of iron. Then this mixture should be ground
together finely and mixed with honey. This will heal aches of the
breast, of the sides, of the liver and of the kidneys if it is eaten
frequently. This will also heal cholera and eases pain in the 'soft'
womb. It comforts the stomach and encourages good digestion.

Folklore ~

Mithridates pronounced
often that rue eaten or
drunk raw will neutralise
poison. For anyone that
eats rue and mint leaves
with a little salt and 2 figs
and 2 acorns and 2 nuts
on an empty stomach,
that day he will dread no
venomous beasts. This
also the weasel teaches,
for when she shall fight
with the adder she will
eat rue first.

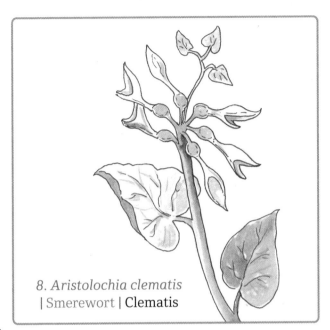

8. Aristolochia clematis
| Smerewort | Clematis

8.

Aristolochia clematis
| Smerewort | Clematis

Smerewort or wodemarch has three varieties. The first is called long because his root is long; the second is called round for the root is round; the third is called in Greek clematis. This is not as strong as the second, which is said to be as round as a radish. All three are hot in the second degree and dry in the first degree.

PRIMARILY

For bites and for venom ~
Make a drink from clematis root and blend with wine and it will heal all venomous bites and destroy poison that has been eaten or drunk and it drives out the afterbirth.

For cold ~
This herb drunk with wine and pepper helps deliver the mother of the afterbirth and from all corruption and filth that might have accumulated, and it will have this effect even if it is only placed at the mouth of the cervix.

For sides or ribs ~
This herb is good for treating coughs and diseases of the sides or ribs. It will ease a chill if the patient feels cold, if it is drunk in well flavoured water or in other liquids that taste equally good.

For nail, thorn or arrow that sticks in a man's body. ~
Grind up this herb and apply as a plaster; it will bring out a nail or thorn or arrow that sticks in a man's body.

For wounds ~
Mix clematis with honey and it will cleanse wounds and heal them.

For teeth ~
Mix with Iris and apply this mixture to the gums; it will keep teeth from rotting and falling out.

For the spleen ~
Drink this herb with vinegar and it will soften the hardness of the spleen.

For the side ~
Drink with hot water or with wine, and it will ease the ache of the side.

For the fevers ~
Drink with water and it will heal fevers.

For the cramp ~
Drink in the same way, and it will be effective against cramp.

For hot gout ~
In the same way it will ease hot gout if it is drunk frequently.

For the falling evil/epilepsy ~
In the same way it will ease the ache of the womb and epilepsy and paralysis as well.

The smoke of this herb will chase away devils and makes young children happy.

For fistulas ~
The root of this herb will heal fistulas effectively, if the area is cleansed and the root is placed securely into the fistula.

For hiccups ~
Drink this herb with water or wine and it will ease hiccupping. It can be used for for the spleen and for any other ailment in a man's body.

The 'long' may do all that I have said that the 'round' may do. But, even so, the long is weaker than the round, if you can't get hold of the round clematis use one and a half times the amount of the long clematis to allow for this difference in strength. A decoction of the long is particularly effective when it is used for bathing or washing. If it is drunk with water it will heal diseases of the spleen - particularly if it is ground up and applied as a poultice.

It will draw out whatever is stuck in a man's body. Also it will heal the 'wicked' humours of the mouth of the womb. Plinius said that a woman that placed this herb to her cervix with beef after she has conceived she shall have a son for this herb forms males in this way.

Mix the round clematis with lime and grind them together - this kills fish; and therefore some men call her 'venom of the earth'.

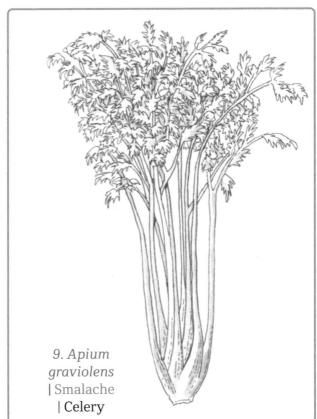

9. Apium
graviolens
| Smalache
| Celery

9.
Apium
graviolens
| Smalache
| Celery

Greeks call this herb
selinon or *solinum*.
It is hot and dry in the
third degree.

PRIMARILY

For swollen eyes and for the stomach ~
Soak the juice of celery with white bread crumbs and plaster it
overnight onto a swollen eye and it will reduce the swelling.
And in the same way it will reduce the swelling of the breasts
and ease the discomfort of the stomach and alleviate flatulence.

To aid urination ~
Eat or drink this herb raw and it will act as a diuretic. A stronger
decoction of this herb is made from the roots; also the seeds of
celery are equally effective if the tea is
drunk frequently.

For poisonous bites and for coughs ~
This herb will help heal venomous bites, the
most effective treatment is to use the seed or
a decoction of the root as a plaster.

In the same way it will ease coughs if you drink celery tea frequently.

For the hard womb ~
Also it will soften the womb and stop vomiting if celery is drunk as a tea.

To restore the colour of the patient ~
Mix celery with a little water and vinegar, taken as a drink this will restore a healthy glow to the patient .

For fevers ~
Eat raw celery on an empty stomach and it will ease fevered conditions, if you drink it with water before the breaking of a fever it will have a cooling effect.

For dropsy/heart failure ~
Drink celery with the juice of fennel and it will help anyone suffering from heart failure or disease in the spleen or swelling of the liver.

For freckles on the face ~
With the juice of celery anoint the freckled face and this will cause the freckles to fade.

For wounds and swellings ~
Mix the juice of celery with meal or wheat flour and the white of an egg to make a plaster, apply this to the area and it will cleanse wounds and swellings if it is used frequently.

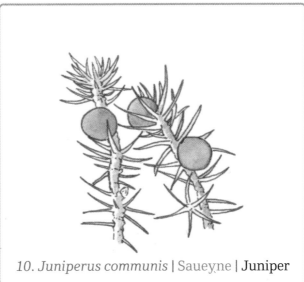

10. Juniperus communis | Saueyne | Juniper

10.
Juniperus communis | Saueyne | Juniper

Juniper is hot and dry in the third degree

PRIMARILY

For wounds or swellings ~
Mix juniper with honey and it will quickly dry a wound or swelling and cleanse it as well.

For a small abscess or boil ~
This plaster will heal a small abscess or boil, which the common people call a swelling.

Juniper will bring on a women's period and cause the dead child in its mother's womb to be born - if it is drunk often with wine or ground up and applied to the mouth of the cervix.

For sickness that is caused by cold ~
Juniper mixed with creosote/creote will make the skin glitter or shine. Juniper will help all sicknesses that are caused by cold if the decoction is drunk with wine or water.

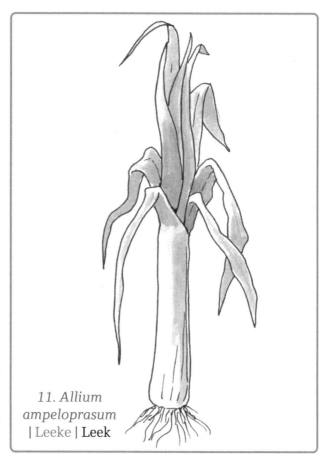

11. *Allium ampeloprasum* | Leeke | Leek

11.
Allium ampelo-prasum | Leeke | Leek

As it is said Hippocrates used leek in many of his medicines

PRIMARILY

Hippocrates that great physician, used the juice of the leek as a drink for people who spit blood, which is known in Greek as ernotoici/blood spitting.

For him that spits blood ~

Make a mixture of 2/3 of frankincense powder or of bile mixed with 1/3 of leek seed and a little myrrh. When all this is mixed together well and soaked in wine it is a healing drink for anyone who spits blood and for nose bleeds.

To staunch nosebleeds ~

The juice of leek will stop nose bleeds if the nostril is covered in leek juice.

This is also good for bleeding from the vagina.

The woman who eats leeks frequently will conceive easily.

For wounds or swellings/tumours/ulcers ~
Mix leek with honey and cover the ulcer or wound with it and it will promote healing.

For dislocation of the head ~
Mix leek juice with hot water, and it will heal the 'dislocation' of the humours of the head and the lungs and also diseases of the breast; and it makes a shrill voice pleasant and soothes the cough that harms the intestines and for everything that has already been mentioned leek juice is very healing.

To ease dysentery ~
Eat leeks and drink wine or drink the juice of leeks mixed with wine and this will make the womb hard. Heat the white of leek in wine and after the first boiling take it out of the wine and boil it in water and give it to the patient to drink; it will stop diarrhoea and make the womb hard, it will act in a similar way if it is soaked in wine and drunk.

For poisonous bites ~
It will destroy the venom of adder bites or of any venomous beast.

For coughs ~
Mix leek juice with woman's milk and this will soothe chronic coughs and be healing to various sicknesses of the lungs.

For the ear ~
Mix the juice of leek with goat's gall or with wine and hold it warm in the ear that aches and it will ease earache.

Leek neutralises the toxins of toadstools .

For the head ~
Mix together two parts of leek juice and the third part of honey, hold it in at the nostril or at the ear and it will soothe headaches.

For the loins ~
As physicians say there is nothing more helpful to the ache of the loins than the juice of leeks drunk with wine.

For swellings ~
Leek or the juice of leek is good for healing fractures and swellings and to soften and relax the hardness of a swelling or of a large deep seated abscess.

For wounds ~
Mix together leek and salt and apply this to a new fresh wound; this will close it quickly.

Eat raw leek and it will relieve drunkenness and act as an aphrodisiac and softens the womb.

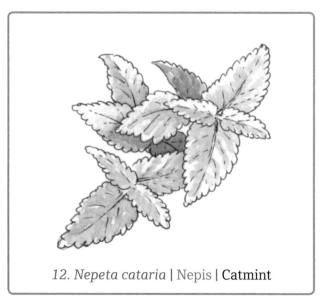

12. Nepeta cataria | Nepis | **Catmint**

12.
Nepeta cataria | Nepis | **Catmint**

Nepys is known in Greek as *calamentum*, and it is dry and hot in the middle of the third degree.

Drink this herb with mead and it will cause sweating.

PRIMARILY

For fever ~
The oil of the decoction of this herb will have a cooling effect, if the body is massaged all over with the oil. The oil also has a warming effect if the patient is cold.

For the disease in the whirlbone (hip) ~
Grind up this herb when it is green and apply it to the thigh as a poultice and it will ease any disease of the hip.

The heat caused by using this herb will inflame the skin and by doing this will ease the disease and aching of the hip.

Mix the juice of this herb into a drink and it will bring on a woman's periods when it is drunk.

For leprosy ~
Elephantitis is a type of leprosy, and it is known by this name because as an elephant is the hugest of all beasts so is this illness the greatest of all illnesses and types of leprosy. Drink catmint at the beginning of this illness with wine, it will prevent the illness developing.

For venom ~
Grind this herb up and apply it to the place that has been bitten by a snake and it will heal it.

For worms of the belly ~
Drink catmint in wine, and it will eliminate venom / poison.

Catmint made into a drink will kill worms in the belly.

Mix the juice of catmint with salt and honey and it will kill worms that are in any area of the body.

If a woman that is with child drinks catmint, it will deliver her of her wherplyng/ deformed child; this herb will have the same effect if it is ground up and placed in the cervix.

For jaundice and tightness of the chest/ shortness of breath.

This herb drunk with wine will cleanse and heal jaundice, shortness of breath and the chincough.

For the liver ~
In the same way it helps ease the pain of the liver.

For the side ~
In the same way it will heal the chronic ache and the pain of the side.

For the cicatrices ~
Grind this herb up and apply it to black cicatrices and it will bring the patient back to the colour that he was before he became ill. But, it is even more effective if it is soaked in wine and then applied externally.

For the stomach ~
Drink the juice of this herb with wine and it will ease the ache and pain of the stomach.

To chase away serpents ~
The smoke of this herb chases serpents out of the house that this herb is burnt in.

For the hiccups ~
It is said that this herb drunk with wine will ease hiccups. It will cause constipation if it is drunk frequently.

There are three types of cat mint: one is like basil, the second is like pennyroyal and is called brotherwort, the third is like mint.

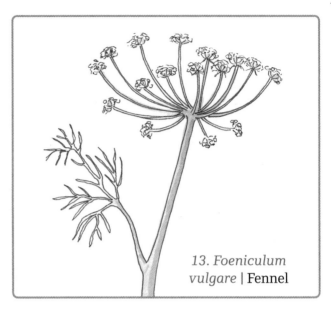

13. *Foeniculum vulgare* | Fennel

13.
Foeniculum vulgare | **Fennel**

Fennel is known in Greek – *maratrum*.

It is hot and dry in the second degree.

PRIMARILY

For venomous bites ~
This herb drunk with wine will heal all types of venomous bites.

For the eyes ~
The adder will eat fennel when her eyes become cloudy and so she regains again her clear sight and therefore this is proof that fennel has a good effect on a person's eyes. Eyes that have been affected by cataracts should be washed with the juice of fennel roots blended with honey and this ointment will clear the dimness of sight caused by this condition.

Wring out the juice of green fennel seed and dry it in the sun and this makes a wonderful medicine for the eyes regardless of the cause of the affliction.

For the ears ~
Hold the juice of fennel in the ear, it will kill all the worms of the ear.

For dropsy (heart failure)and the lungs ~
Soak fennel in wine and drink it, it will reduce the swelling caused by heart failure - this causes fluid retention either in the legs or head and chest. It will also heal poisonous bites and heal the lungs and the liver as well .

To encourage breast milk production ~
To produce plentiful breast milk eat and drink fennel herb and seed.

For the kidneys and the bladder ~
Infuse in wine or water the roots of fennel and this decoction will heal the ache of the kidneys and the pains of the bladder.

For to piss/promote urination ~
Eat fennel or drink the juice of it and it will ease any restriction in urination and bring on women's periods. Or grind fennel and bind it to the penis/pubic region/groin and it will also heal this area.

For vomiting ~
Drink the juice of fennel with wine and it will stop vomiting.

For kidneys ~
The root of fennel infused in hot water is excellent medicine for the kidneys.

For the stomach ~
The juice of fennel drunk with wine cools the heat of the stomach.

For a man's penis ~
The root of fennel soaked in wine and applied to the penis helps ease the ache of that area. This decoction also helps if it is drunk or used as a bath for the penis. It has a similar effect if the root is infused in oil and this is applied to the penis.

Swellings ~
Crush and mix the juice of fennel with oil and apply to the place that is swollen through a blow or any other cause: this will reduce the swelling and it is equally effective if fennel is crushed with vinegar and a plaster is made of the mixture and applied to the affected area.

For to keep a man long young/for eternal youth ~
A decoction of fennel drunk regularly will make old men seem young.

Fennel seed drunk with wine acts as an aphrodisiac.

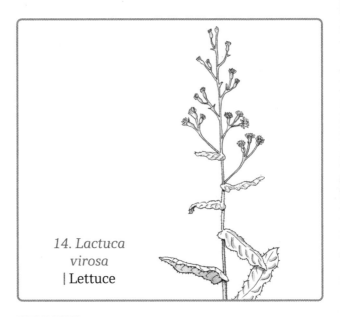

*14. Lactuca
virosa
| Lettuce*

14.

Lactuca virosa | **Lettuce**

Lettuce is cold and right moist, and therefore this herb heals many diseases if it is eaten and also if it is ground up and used as a plaster.

PRIMARILY

For the stomach and sleep ~
Lettuce is good for the stomach. It encourages you to sleep well and also works as a laxative. For the best effects eat and drink lettuce after it has been infused first rather than eaten raw.

For dreams and haemorrhaging ~
The seed of lettuce drunk with wine prevents vivid and frightening dreams and also staunches haemorrhaging of the womb.

For the stomach ~
For the stomach lettuce is best eaten raw and unwashed.

For nocturnal emissions of sperm ~
He who often suffers from nocturnal emissions, if he eats this herb and drinks the juice of it will soon be saved from such events.

For a nursing mother ~
A nursing mother who eats lettuce will have a plentiful supply of milk, but some say that if you eat a lot of this herb you will go blind due to eating excessive amounts of it.

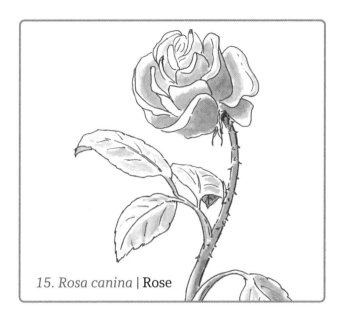

15. Rosa canina | Rose

15.
Rosa canina | Rose

The rose may well be called the flower of flowers because she outdoes all other flowers with her beauty and fragrance and the many varieties of her colours.

The red rose is known as rosa canina, another wild rose is known in Rome as *saliunca*.

The rose is dry and cold in the first degree.

PRIMARILY

For diarrhoea ~
Drink the juice of roses and it will stop the flux that is known as diarrhoea.

Rose juice also eases heavy periods.

For wounds ~
A plaster made of roses will dry rotten/boggy wounds.

Constantinus says that the rose is hot and dry; this is said of the wild rose that I am familiar with. Of the other, that is to say garden roses I will give you some more information.

The rose not only heals through her scent and her beauty but she is also useful in a variety of medicines.

A primary use is in the treatment of holy fire (ergot poisoning); the rose eases the pain of holy fire if it is ground up and laid upon the affected area.

Similarly if the stomach is too hot or the intestines are affected in the area around the heart, crush the rose petals and apply as a plaster to the affected area and it will reduce the heat.

A bath of these roses soaked in wine or drunk will ease bleeding from the uterus.

For the womb ~
The juice of roses is good for a variety of ailments of the womb.

For the mouth ~
The powder of dried roses eases many irritations of the mouth.

For the gums ~
The powder of the rose flower rubbed on to the lips or mixed with honey is good for cracked lips and sore gums.

For fierce heat ~
Rose will cool all types of overheating if the fresh petals are ground up and applied to the area or drunk in wine.

For the womb and the stomach ~
From the rose is made rose oil, which heals many afflictions and especially if it is drunk it will soften the womb and cool the immoderate heat of the stomach.

For the head ~
With this oil wash, bathe or anoint the head to ease headaches and the heat of the head.

For wounds ~
This oil will also help clean filthy wounds and encourage good flesh to grow in deep wounds, particularly if mixed with a strong vinegar.

For burns ~
And in the same way it is cooling and healing for burns and scalds.

For toothache ~
If you hold this oil in your mouth for a long time it will ease toothache.

This oil will ease the itch of the membranes within if it is placed around the area, and this oil is useful for many complaints of the vulva and vagina.

Different people have a variety of ways of making this oil but the Greek clerk Pallidus wrote down the way that he recommends making it: take the red petals of the rose (The Damascus Rose) - one ounce of petals to a pound of oil. Put all this into a glass jar and stand it in the sun for seven days, or you can hang it near the fire or in the sun for 15 days. After this time strain it through a clean cloth and keep the oil to use in various medicines.

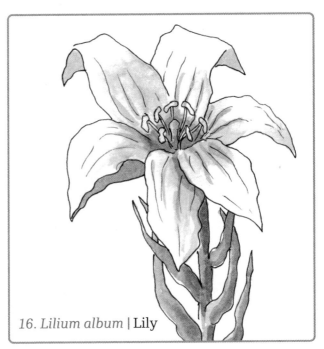

16. *Lilium album* | Lily

16.
Lilium album | Lily

After the gentle and golden roses rightfully what should follow next but the silvery lily. In many cases the lily is also as useful to man as the rose is for medicines.

PRIMARILY

For scalds ~
The lily root roasted under coals and afterwards grated small and mixed with cumin oil, will heal burns and scalds, but it will do even better if you include some rose oil as well.

Lily root mixed in the same way and applied to the vulva makes the hard womb soft.

For sinews and limbs and venomous bites ~
A plaster made of soaked lily leaves helps the sinews that have been drawn together (shortened by injury) and relaxes them. In the same way it helps the limbs that have been bent through injury. It also heals adder bites.

For toadstool poisoning ~
Lily root soaked in wine and drunk neutralises the poison of toadstools.

To draw out nails or thorns from a body ~
Crush lily roots and infuse them in wine and make a plaster of this mixture and it will draw out the nail, thorn or stick or arrow stuck in the feet or elsewhere. This plaster should be left in place for three days.

It is said that lily root soaked in pig grease or in sheep tallow will make hair grow on the limbs that have been burnt.

For the spleen ~
Men say that lily roots soaked in wine and drunk, purge accumulated blood from the womb and in a similar way it supports the spleen. It also heals the cervix, and brings on women's periods. All this will be achieved if it is soaked in old wine and applied as a plaster.

For wounds ~
Lily roots crushed well and mixed with honey is medicine for broken or cut or hurt sinews/ligaments/tendons.

There is nothing better for drying up wounds than the juice squeezed out of lily leaves mixed with vinegar and soaked in honey. To make this mixture take five parts of lily juice and 2 parts of vinegar and honey. Another book says that the honey and vinegar should make up 4 parts and the juice the fifth part. Either of these recipes will dry up both old and new wounds and heal them cleanly.

This same juice will heal wounds and cleanse them.

For the face ~
Lily roots soaked and ground up and mixed with creote or with wax and butter will smooth out all the wrinkles of the face and get rid of all the freckles of the skin if this ointment is used frequently.

For leprous or scrofula conditions ~
This same ointment will heal the condition that is known in Latin as lichene or variole and in English, measles. This ointment will also cleanse the face of the black scrofula.

Crush the lily leaves and apply the juice to the cervix to soften it. This juice will cause sweating if it is applied liberally all over the body.

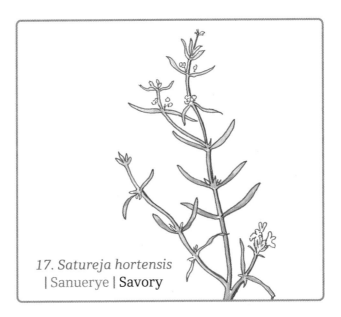

17. Satureja hortensis
| Sanuerye | **Savory**

17. Satureja hortensis | Sanuerye | Savory

Among the herbs that Putagoras discusses, he has the highest praise for savory.

Savory is both hot and dry in the first degree.

PRIMARILY

Savory draws out and thins sticky mucous and burns the skin. So great is her might and heat, but there is more value in savoury seed than there is in the herb.

For the stone ~

Savoury seed when eaten helps you to think clearly and sharpens the wit and dissolves kidney stones and eases urination, and it brings on women's periods.

For the head ~

Savoury seed ground up small and blended with warm water, held and rolled about the pallet of the mouth whilst facing the sun will cleanse the noxious mucous from the head.

It is good to eat or drink the seed if you suffer from sneezing, because it eases congestion of the head.

For the stomach ~

When eaten, the seed comforts the stomach and eases shortness of breath.

For adder bites ~

This seed ground up finely with vinegar and laid upon adder bites will heal them.

This seed when eaten neutralises the poison of toadstools and prevents the poison from causing any digestive discomfort.

For the head ~

I have already said that savoury and her seed are both very
hot, to such a degree that they will burn and break the skin. But
without any doubt such a hotness and dryness is very useful in
many situations for through such a heat thick mucus and toxins
of the head will be dried up. Also will the humour be dried up
that falls from the head to the eyes and even that humour that
falls down from the head to the lungs and causes illness.

For the stomach ~

This will also heal many sicknesses of the stomach and coughs
due to the heat and drying effect of savoury seed.

For sciatica ~

This heating herb will also draw out the old ache and the disease
of the thighs and the bladder, which is known in Greek as
sciatica.

For the spleen and the liver ~

This mixture will also ease the hard swellings of the spleen and
liver. This mixture is very healing for many chronic ailments. To
make a poultice of savoury seeds for the most efficacious effect
I will say how Menemacus commanded to make it. (Other
physicians may make it differently).

Take savoury seeds and grind them well in a mortar, add three
parts of crumbs of white bread and add to this dried figs and
honey and vinegar, after this it depends on the condition, for the
more dried figs and honey the stronger is the savoury, but the
more bread you put in with the vinegar, the weaker is the plaster
of savoury. I ask you to take this information seriously, because
I have proved how effective this mixture is in many cases but be
careful only to use it on old and chronic sores and not on open
wounds.

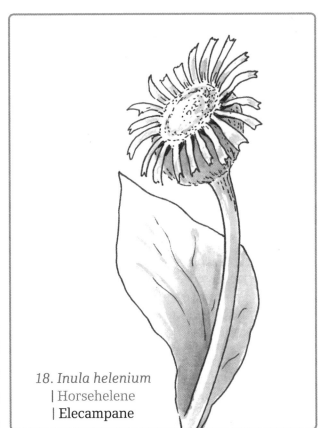

18. *Inula helenium*
| Horsehelene
| Elecampane

18.
Inula helenium
| Horsehelene
| Elecampane

Horsehelene is called henula and commonly elena, and physicians call her elenium. All men know well the shape of this herb.

PRIMARILY

This herb is moist and cold in the first degree and hot in the second degree. A decoction of this herb brings on a women's periods.

For to piss/to encourage urination ~
This herb enables you to urinate easily and also it will deliver a child that is dead in the mother's womb and also softens the womb that is congested.

For the thigh ~
The root of this herb ground up and applied to the thigh as a poultice will heal the pain in the hip known as sciatica.

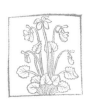

For the kidneys ~

The leaves of this herb soaked in pyment (wine infused with honey and spices) and placed over the kidneys will heal aching and the disease of the kidneys which is called nephritis.

For coughs ~

A powder of the root eaten with honey will soothe coughs and in the same way this medicine will help anyone who has the 'chincost'.

Orthonoyci is when he can draw in as much air as he puts out. Asmaticus is that he breaths out more air than he breaths in. Disnoicus is when he can take more air in than he can breathe out. And all these three conditions cause coughing but in different ways.

For people that have been injured ~

Mix the juice of this herb with the juice of rue in equal measures, soaked together this makes a valuable medicine if it is drunk by people who have been injured.

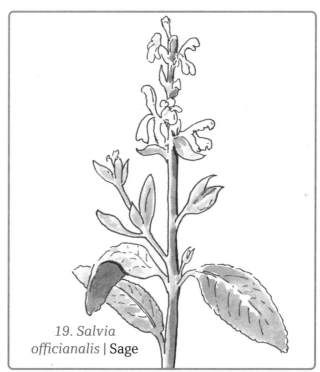

19. Salvia officianalis | Sage

19.
Salvia officianalis | Sage

Sage is known in Latin as salgea and saluia

PRIMARILY

For the liver ~
Sage drunk with mulsa wine helps heal all the diseases of the liver, and in the same way will deliver a woman of a child that is dead in her body and brings on women's periods and enables a person to 'piss fast', (urinate easily).

For venomous bites and wounds ~
Sage ground up and mixed with salt cures venomous bites and stops the bleeding of new wounds.

For coughs ~
The juice of sage drunk with wine will ease a chronic cough and aches of the side.

The wine that sage is soaked in will alleviate itching of the vagina and of a man's penis if they are frequently washed with this mixture.

The juice of sage will make grey hair black if it is applied frequently in the heat of the sun.

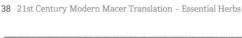

20.
Hyssopus officinalis
| Isope
| Hyssop

20. *Hyssopus officinalis* | Isope | Hyssop

Hyssop is dry and hot in the third degree

The decoction of hyssop with honey and dried figs eaten or drunk will help heal coughs or catarrh.

PRIMARILY

For hoarseness ~
This decoction helps anyone that is hoarse or who has a lung disease.

For worms ~
This decoction destroys worms in the belly.

For the breast ~
If there is any mucus or 'down falling of humours' from the head to the breast which is likely to bring on a cough the remedy is the same decoction as above, drunk frequently.

To treat all diseases as mentioned before; take some powdered hyssop and blend with honey to make a valuable medicine.

For the womb ~
Green hyssop ground up and mixed with oxymel - a drink made from vinegar and honey, two parts vinegar to three parts honey. Drink this and it will ease the hard womb and make it soft.

In the same way it eliminates noxious wind and the vicious and 'gletty' phlegm, it works even more effectively if you add cardamom (kerson) to the mixture.

A portion of fresh or dried hyssop drunk with wine will make a person's face 'well coloured'.

For dropsy/heart failure ~
Blend hyssop with dried figs and with nitrum, this applied liberally over a swollen spleen will reduce the swelling. It also helps with reducing the fluid that accumulates in dropsy (heart failure).

For swellings ~
Hyssop drunk with wine relaxes the intestines that have been in spasm and also helps reduce abdominal swellings.

For toothache ~
Frequently wash aching teeth in vinegar that has had hyssop soaking in it and this will relieve toothache.

For ringing in the ears (tinnitus) ~
Burn hyssop to ease the ringing in the ears.

Soaked hyssop laid over the eyes makes them bright and removes all cloudiness from the eyes.

For jaundice ~
In the same way breathing in the smoke from burnt hyssop will heal jaundice.

For the ears ~
It is said a blend of soaked hyssop and oil of roses held in the ear will ease earache.

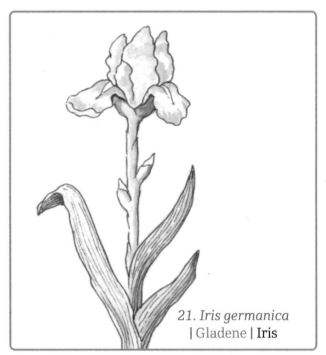

21. *Iris germanica*
| Gladene | Iris

21.
Iris germanica | Gladene | Iris

Gladene in English is called *iris* in Latin, its flowers have colours like the rainbow.

This herb is hot and dry in the second degree but it is the root of this herb that has the greatest value.

PRIMARILY

Take the root of this herb and cut it into round gobbettes or discs and then hang the discs on a thread without letting any of them touch each other. If you want to dry them effectively hang the string of root discs in a dry place in the shade, if you don't do this then they won't dry even if you leave them for a whole year.

For the mouth ~

Drink the powder of this in wine and it will ease coughs and give you a well flavoured mouth. It also sweetens the breath and removes any rottenness - if there is any lurking within hurting and aggravating the intestines.

For cholera ~

This powder drunk with mulsa wine heals the cholera. Mulsa is a drink made of honey and water, 8 parts water and the ninth part honey.

For veins ~

Mix this powder with vinegar and drink it, it will ease any problems of the womb and it is good for the veins.

For the spleen ~
This powder is medicinal to anyone that has a disease of the spleen and to anyone who has been badly chilled or hurt with cold if it is drunk with wine.

In the same way it will bring on a woman's period if it is slow or late.

For the womb ~
A decoction of iris roots will soften the hardness of the cervix if the area is washed and massaged frequently, and if it is also drunk by the patient as well.

For sciatica ~
This decoction put in the rectum as an enema will ease the pain that is called sciatica.

Iris roots and honey mixed together make a medicine which if it is placed into the vagina will encourage the expulsion of the afterbirth.

For wounds ~
The powder of iris roots mixed with honey will dry up wounds and cover the area with good clean flesh, it causes the flesh to regenerate.

For the face ~
Take two parts of powdered iris root and the third part of powdered hellebore root and mix these powders together with honey, apply this to the face and your face will be cleansed of freckles, pockets and welks.

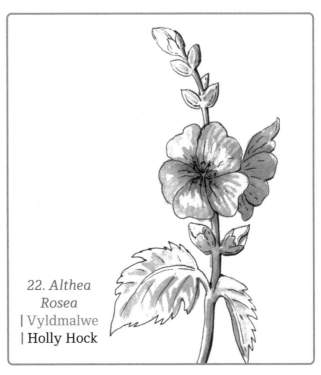

22. Althea
     Rosea
| Vyldmalwe
| Holly Hock

22.
*Althea
Rosea*
| Vyldmalwe
| **Hollyhock**

Vyldmalwe is called
holly hock and in Latin
we call her *althea*, some
men call her the
wild mallow.

PRIMARILY

For wounds ~

The flower of this herb soaked in mulsa cleans wounds, you can drink this mixture and make a poultice of it.

It will spread or move throughout the body and destroy worms also helping to ease aching eyes.

For bruises ~

In the same way it is said that it is good for bruises.

The root soaked and afterwards mixed well with pig fat and turpentine is said to heal swellings of the cervix and all other aches or diseases of this area and generally relax the tissues of this area.

For large deep seated abscesses ~
It breaks up and softens hard abscesses.

For all these ailments a decoction of this herb will help if the place that needs healing is frequently bathed or anointed with the warmed mixture.

For the bloody dysentery ~
A decoction of this root drunk with wine will ease the bloody dysentery and rapidly expels the afterbirth.

For the bladder ~
This is good for anyone that spits blood. It will also dissolve bladder stones and will help other bladder ailments.

For spots ~
Grind the seed of this herb and mix with vinegar and add to it olive oil and this ointment will heal spots and acne.

For poisoning ~
This herb will destroy any venom if it is drunk with pusca.

For wounds ~
This herb soaked and afterwards ground up with honey will heal hollow wounds and fill them with good flesh if it is used frequently.

For swellings ~
A plaster made of the leaves of this herb soaked in oil will soften all hardness and ease all stiffness.

For venomous bites ~
The ashes of this herb will heal all venomous bites if they are applied often to the affected area.

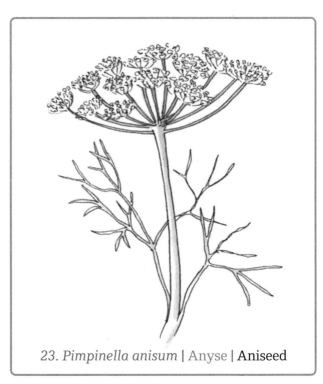

23. *Pimpinella anisum* | Anyse | **Aniseed**

23.
Pimpinella anisum | Anyse | Aniseed

Aniseed is hot and dry in the second degree.

PRIMARILY

For headache ~
The flower of aniseed soaked in oil and bound to the head will ease headaches.

For the stomach ~
A decoction of aniseed drunk frequently will increase breast milk in nursing mothers. It will heal diseases of the stomach, take three ciatus of warm aniseed decoction and this will open the stomach allowing noxious wind to be released and it also eases vomiting and nausea.

Ciatus is the quantity that half an egg shell can hold'.

To encourage urination ~
This same drink will encourage urination and ease any obstructions that might prevent this.

This drink will help the cervix relax particularly if it is used in a warm bath.

For the womb ~
Aniseed ground up and drunk in warm water will help ease the ache of the intestines and of the womb and helps digestion because it acts as a gentle laxative.

Aniseed drunk regularly prevents the way of child getting (conception) and dries up the humours of the seed within the body thereby preventing conception.

For wounds and swellings ~
The ashes of aniseed will abrade away the damaged flesh that develops in wounds and it cleans the swellings that creep from one place to another and it also purges foul wounds.

If the little 'gobet' in the mouth that is known as the uvula is swollen the ashes of aniseed put in with a finger or applied using a syringe will heal it quickly.

It is said that the ashes of the root are quicker to work than the ashes of the herb.

For the penis ~
These ashes will heal swellings and especially those of a man's penis.

For hiccups ~
Roast aniseed seed and breathe in the smoke to stop hiccups.

For the eyes ~
Aniseed roasted and ground up and applied to the eyes will have a cooling effect.

For haemorrhoids ~
Aniseed roasted and applied to haemorrhoids will heal them and dissolve the hard swelling in the ear or anywhere else.

For cold and for the head ~
Steep aniseed flour in oil and it will be medicinally effective, warming and driving out cold and it will often stop headaches and reduce swellings of the veins and has an overall warming effect.

24. *Stachys betonica*
| Betoyne
| Wood Betony

24. *Stachys betonica* | Betoyne | Wood Betony

Betoyne is known in Greek as *castron*.

It is used primarily for treating 'the stone'. Betony if drunk as a tea acts as a diuretic - 'makes a body for to piss well and putteth out the stone'.

Betony drunk with wine will help heal haemoptysis (one who spits blood).

PRIMARILY

For the throat and neck ~
Betony pulverised and applied as a plaster will heal aches of the throat and neck.

For the ears ~
The juice of betony blended with oil of roses and dropped into the ears will heal many sores and sicknesses (of the ears).

For the nose ~
To stop a nose bleed. This herb bruised well and put into the nostril will stop blood running out of the nose.

For empyema ~
The powder of betony soaked in honey will help the sicknesses that physicians call empicos. It will also soothe coughs.

For fevers ~
This powder drunk with wine will cool fevers .

For the head ~
Betony bruised and applied to the head will heal fractures of the head.

For the eyes ~
Betony leaves soaked and applied to the eyes will soothe various sores of the eyes. Betony eaten or drunk will dry watering eyes.

A plaster made of betony leaves well pulverised will heal eyes that have been hurt through a stroke. Apply the plaster and lie still all night.

Take betony and also the same amount of rue and eat and drink this mixture and it might heal cataracts.

The juice of betony drunk with warm water will cleanse and ease painful suffering from an abscess or ulceration. Also this same drink will heal sores of the breast.

For the spleen ~
A decoction of betony helps both the spleen and the liver.

For the kidneys ~
Take 4oz of betony and three ciatus of old wine, 27 peppercorns well 'brayed', ground in a mortar, place all this together and drink it and this will heal all ailments of the kidneys.

For the womb ~
1 dragm of betony drunk with 2 ciatus of warm water or wine will ease the ache of the womb.

For toothache ~
Betony juice held in the mouth for a long time will relieve toothache.

For the cough ~
Betony eaten with honey will ease coughs and bring on delayed periods

For fevers ~
2 dragm plantain with 1 dragm of betony ground together and drunk in warm water before the cold chills develop will ease the fever (ague quotidian).

For dropsy/ heart failure ~
1oz of betony infused in a ciatus of hot water will help anyone who has heart failure if it is drunk frequently.

The powder of betony roots drunk in mulsa wine eliminates stones and the 'noxious humours' in a similar way to hellebore.

As a purgative ~
Plinius's recipe; take 4 dragms of betony root and give it as a drink in mulsa or vino passum to ease constipation. *Vinum passum* is a wine that is squeezed out of dried grapes, that is to say of such grapes that have been laid out in the sun for to dry somewhat and are stiffened in the same way as hay.

For adder bites ~
In the same way it will heal adder bites.

For venom ~
Betony neutralises all types of venom

For drunkenness ~
If you eat betony you will not become drunk - during that day.

For jaundice ~
1 oz of betony drunk in wine heals jaundice and infused in mulsa it will bring on women's periods.

For the stomach ~
The powder of betony equivalent to a bean in weight, eaten after supper with honey, helps the stomach digest meat.

Menemacus said 'include this herb in all medicines for the stomach as it is the most appropriate and profitable herb to the stomach out of all herbs'.

For evil drinks ~
Plinius said that anyone who carries with him this herb will not be harmed by any 'evil' drinks.

For good colour ~
And he also said that this herb drunk often with wine will give a person a healthy colour.

Folklore ~
As Plinius said: if around a group of serpents a circle of green betony is laid, they shall not go over or under this circle nor pass out of it, but there over the course of time they will bite and beat each other with their tails until they are all dead.

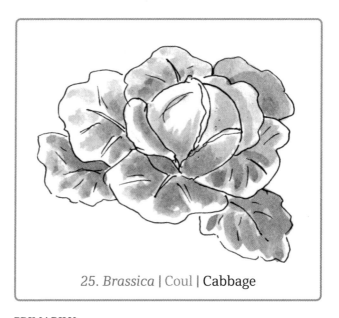

25. Brassica | Coul | Cabbage

25. *Brassica* | Coul | Cabbage

Coul in Greek is known as *brassica*. It is a common herb, but despite this it is a very useful herb medicinally and will heal many illnesses. Caton says that six hundred years before the time that physicians wrote about the medicines used in Rome, the Romans used cabbage as an important medicine.

Cabbage is cold and dry in the first degree.

PRIMARILY

For wounds ~
As the same Caton says, cabbage ground up and applied as a plaster will heal wounds, not only new, but also old, chronic conditions.

For cancers ~
The same Caton says that cabbage will heal cancers. He suggests that the place is first washed with warm wine or water, and then take raw cabbage and grind it up and apply the fresh cabbage mixture as a poultice, twice daily.

For gout of the foot ~
Caton instructs us to take barley meal, cabbage and rue and coriander with a little salt and grind all this together to make a plaster and then apply it to the affected area.

For arthritis ~
This same plaster will also heal the pains of the toes and of the joints, which is called arthritis.

For fistulas and for painful wounds ~
This plaster will heal fistulas and that disease that is known as subluxation - dislocation of joints, and many other painful wounds if it is applied to the area.

This same Caton says that if cabbage is eaten regularly, it is a very good treatment for diseases of the ligaments, if the cabbage is bruised and the affected area washed with the juice.

The juice will also heal children if the affected area is often washed with the cabbage juice.

For the eyes ~

Crisippus says of the virtues of this herb that all physicians agree on is that cabbage cleanses and makes eyes bright in people who eat it often as a green plant; and in the same way it helps increase breast milk production and brings on women's periods. It also helps protect the stomach.

It is said that if the cabbage is well cooked and then eaten it will make you constipated and cabbage half cooked will have a laxative effect.

For the spleen ~

Dip cabbage in vinegar and eat it raw, and it will reduce the swelling of the spleen.

The seed of the cabbage will deliver a woman of her dead child from her womb.

For the fever ~

Take vinegar and old pig fat and cabbage and grind them well together. Then heat all this together and add to it oil of roses as much as you think is enough. This decoction reduces the great heat of the fever, if you apply it to the stomach and other areas that are hot.

For the leper ~

Take whole alum and sharp vinegar and cabbages. Grind this mixture up so that they are all incorporated together. With this ointment you might ease the lepers pain. If you anoint the place frequently with this ointment it will prevent hairs from falling out - baldness.

For testicles ~

Physicians say that this ointment helps swollen testicles and other various sores that affect the genitalia, and this cure will be even more effective if you include soaked beans into the mixture.

For the hot gout ~
Grind cabbage with fenugreek and vinegar and apply this mixture to the toes that ache and it will help the pain known as arthritis; therefore it will also help ease the pain of gout.

For aches and pains ~
The ash of cabbage well ground with old pig fat and applied as a plaster will help ease the old aches both of the side and of the thigh; though this is a foul medicine it is effective.

For the womb ~
The seed of cabbage drunk in vinegar will destroy the noxious beasties of the womb.

For the mouth ~
Take dry cabbage roots and burn them, take the powder or the ash, put it under that part of the mouth that is known as the uvula, this mixture will ease any swelling in this area.

For laryngitis ~
Physicians say that it is good for anyone that has lost their voice to chew cabbage well and gargle with the juice.

For anyone that is melancholy cabbage will produce an increased blood supply to the head and generally act as a tonic.

For the head ~
The juice of cabbage held in at the nostril will clear the head.

For drunkenness ~
He that eats cabbage first in the morning, will not feel drunk that day.

For the mouth ~
Mellicus says that a cabbage root that has never touched the earth after it was pulled up out of the ground, hung about the neck, should keep and heal the uvula of the mouth from all ailments that might afflict it.

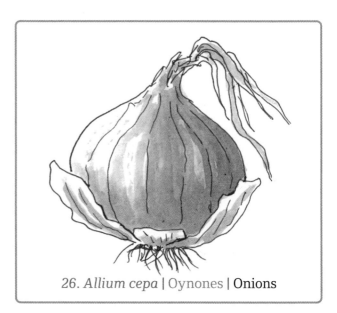

26. Allium cepa | Oynones | **Onions**

26. *Allium cepa* | Oynones | Onions

Onions are good; but it seems that not all physicians agree in the effect that they have, for Dioscorides says that they cause the head to swell and makes you feel ill if you eat raw onion. Galen says that onions are not good for melancholy folk, but to phlegmatic folks he says that they are very good. Asclepinus says that they are good and particularly for the stomach.

PRIMARILY

Onions are good and hot in the fourth degree and moist in the second degree.

Asclepius says that onions make anyone who eats them look well and healthy.

For long life ~
Any one that eats onions first thing each day, shall live long without any sickness.

For dog bites ~
Physicians say that onions will heal dog bites if they are applied to the bite, but first they must be ground up well and mixed with honey and vinegar. Another method is to warm onions in honey and wine and then use the mixture as a poultice; leave for three days then remove the plaster.

For snake bites ~
Diascorides says that onions, salt and rue should be applied to snake bites, for swift healing

For the ear ~
The juice of onions mixed with woman's milk and held in the ear will ease earache.

For laxative ~
All physicians know well that onions act as a laxative.

For dumb men ~
The juice of onions mixed with water and drunk will help anyone who has an inflammation that has made him dumb.

For the head ~
The juice of onions inhaled through the nostril will eliminate noxious humours of the head.

Onions eaten and drunk bring on a women's periods when they are late.

For feet ~
The juice of onions will heal fractures of the feet or the hard skin on the soles of the feet, if you blend it together with hens grease and apply it to the affected area.

For tooth ache ~
Physicians say that anyone who rubs and washes his teeth with the juice of onions daily, will not suffer from tooth ache.

Onions eaten with bread will ease any swellings of the mouth.

For bloody dysentery ~
Soaked onions dipped in oil and eaten stops the griping pain of the bloody dysentery.

For coughs ~
Onion seed decoction drunk frequently helps soothe coughs.

To cure baldness ~
With onions ground up small you might restore hair to the head, if you apply the mixture frequently to the place where the hairs have been falling away.

Onions cleanse the stink and the foul odour of the mouth.

For haemorrhoids ~
Onions ground up small and applied as a plaster eases the discomfort of haemorrhoids.

For the eyes ~
Onion juice with honey mixed together cleans the eyes and make them bright if they are often washed with the mixture.

For freckles ~
Onion juice melded with vinegar is known to remove spots or freckles if it is applied frequently to the area.

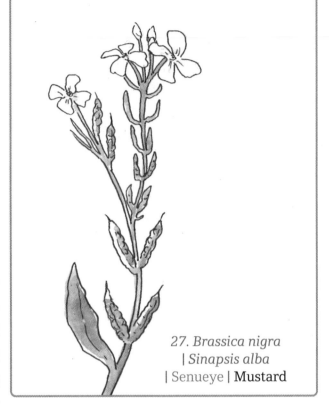

27. *Brassica nigra*
| *Sinapsis alba*
| Senueye | **Mustard**

27.
Brassica nigra | Sinapsis alba | Senueye | Mustard

Among the herbs that Putagoras praised, he gives the first and highest praise to mustard.

Mustard is both hot and dry in the first degree.

PRIMARILY

Mustard draws out and thins the viscous humours and burns the skin. So great is the heat, and mustard seed is stronger than the herb.

For the stone ~
Mustard seed when eaten sharpens the wit and stirs the womb and breaks the kidney stone and acts as a diuretic, and it brings on a woman's periods.

For the head ~
Mustard seed ground up finely and mixed with warm water held and rolled about the pallet of the mouth will cleanse the noxious 'fumes' of the head.

It is good to eat or drink the seed to cause sneezing, because it eases the tightness of the head.

For the stomach –
This seed when eaten comforts the stomach and eases shortness of breath.

For adder bites –
This seed ground up small with vinegar and laid upon adder bites will heal them.

This seed when eaten destroys the poison of toadstools and prevents the venom from troubling the intestines.

For the head –
It is said previously that mustard and its seed are both known to be very hot, such that they will burn and burst the skin. But without any doubt such a hotness is appropriate in many situations, for through such a heat noxious humours are drawn out of the head and dried up. Mustard also dries up the liquid that falls from the head to the eyes and also phlegm that collects in the lungs which can cause chronic illnesses.

For the stomach –
This heat will also heal many sicknesses of the stomach and also coughs.

For sciatica –
This heat will draw out the old ache and the disease of the thighs, which is known as sciatica.

For the spleen and the liver –
This herb will also soften the hard swellings of the spleen and of the liver, and ease many other old conditions.

To learn how to make a plaster of this herb or of its seed is a good idea, physicians make this plaster in different ways, therefore I will tell you how Menemacus made it. Take some mustard seeds and grind them well in a mortar: make up the third part of white bread crumbs: take them and add to them dry figs, honey and vinegar, after that it depends on the quantity that is sufficient, the more figs and honey you use the sharper is the mustard but the more bread and vinegar you use, the weaker the plaster. I admonish and counsel that you appreciate the value of this confection, for I have proved its full value in many causes, but never the less do not apply it to all sores, but only onto long standing old sores. (Never on to an open wound).

As with savory on page 33.

28. Piper album | White Pepper

28.
Piper album | **White Pepper**

White pepper or white senuey is known in Latin as eruca.

It is hot and dry in the middle degree; but it is not as dry as it is hot.

This herb when eaten helps with digestion

This herb when eaten or drunk will enable the eater to urinate easily.

This herb when eaten will ease children's coughs.

PRIMARILY

For spots and freckles ~
This herb ground small with honey and applied to the skin will heal the spots on the face and clear it of freckles.

For broken bones ~
The root of this herb soaked and ground up small and then applied to the fracture will heal broken bones.

For strokes ~
The seed of this herb ground up and drunk with wine will heal all types of strokes.

For spots ~
This herb ground up with ox gall and applied to the area will heal all black spots.

Meat cooked with this herb or its seed has a good flavour.

The seed eaten or drunk causes sexual arousal as lecherous people confirm as do many poets.

White pepper is particularly good when eaten with lettuce, the heat from the pepper tempers the coolness of the lettuce.

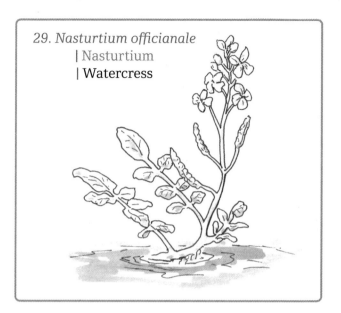

29. Nasturtium officianale
| Nasturtium
| Watercress

29.
Nasturtium officianale
| **Nasturtium**
| **Watercress**

This is hot and dry in the middle of the third degree.

PRIMARILY

This herb if it is eaten frequently will reduce lechery by drying the seed of the eater in a similar way to rue.

For boils and carbuncles ~

This herb ground up small and mixed well with sour dough will heal a boil/small abscess, if it is well plastered to the affected area. This medicine will heal the sore that is known as a carbuncle, for this plaster will make it come to a head, release its pus and heal thereby relieving the patient of the pain of the carbuncle.

For warts ~

This same plaster will get rid of warts.

Wash the balding/thinning head with the juice of this herb and thin hair will not fall out.

For toothache ~

Hold the juice onto the side that the tooth aches and it will ease the tooth ache, the seed of this herb is stronger than the herb.

For venom ~

This seed drunk with wine will deliver a woman of her child, if it is dead in her belly. It kills the worms of the womb, and it will destroy all venoms and it is said that the smell of the seeds of this herb when heated on the coals of a fire will drive away poisonous snakes.

This seed drunk frequently with vinegar will have a soothing effect on the spleen.

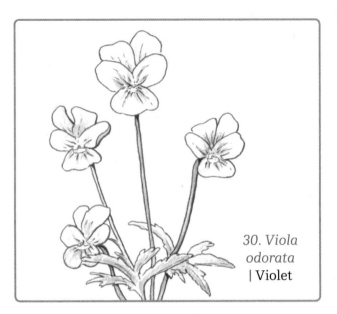

30. Viola odorata | Violet

30.

Viola odorata | **Violet**

Neither the colours of roses or lilies can surpass the violet, neither in beauty, neither in strength or virtue, neither in odour.

It is said that violet is moist and cold in the 4th degree. Of violet there are three varieties - white, black and purple.

PRIMARILY

For heat ~
Violet soothes and refreshes the places that have been inflamed and hot, if it is pulped and applied as a plaster.

For the head ~
Violet eases headaches if it is drunk or applied to the head and bandaged up.

For the groin ~
Water that violet is soaked in is good for the diseases of the groin, if the area is often washed and bathed with the violet water.

For the falling evil/epilepsy ~
It is said that the purple violet helps and heals epilepsy especially in children if it is drunk with water.

For the eyes ~
Crush violet with myrrh and saffron and apply this plaster to swellings on the eye and it will heal it.

For swellings of the head ~
Grind violets with honey and vinegar and apply to head injuries.

With the water that violet is soaked in, wash and bathe often the womb, and it will ease any swellings .

For the ears ~
Mix violets with wax and apply often to the cracks of the ears, which are known as fissures.

Violet seed drunk with wine will bring on a woman's period.

For the spleen ~
Violet roots ground up and blended with vinegar dry the spleen if it is drunk or applied to the area.

For gout ~
It is said that in this same way it might cure and heal hot gout.

For the stomach ~
Drink green violet infusion or the juice of it and the red cholera in the stomach will be healed.

For the sides ~
A drink made from violets soaked in fresh water will heal all the sicknesses that come of the 'cholera rubea' or of blood in the tender and soft sides or in the lungs and the coughs of children and shortness of breath.

For ears and the head ~
As you make oil of roses so make oil of violets, this is helpful in many ways, it will heal the ache of the ears and tinnitus, if it is put in them, and it also eases headaches.

For worms ~
Hold in or drink this oil or anoint the womb and it will kill any worms that are present.

For the body ~
It cools the body.

Dandruff ~
Rub the scalp with this oil and it will heal the scaly dust known as dandruff.

For a fractured skull ~
If the skull or the brain be broken or bowed, so that the patient may not speak, crush this violet and get him to drink it in wine. Afterwards, if the right side of his head hurts, crush the violet and bind it to the sole of his left foot; if it is the reverse, do the reverse, after a while the bone will begin to heal and the same day the patient will speak as normal to the physician.

For haemorrhaging of the womb ~
The root of the white violet will staunch the haemorrhaging of the womb.

A wound, whether old or new heals quickly if violet juice is mixed with liquorice and applied to the affected area.

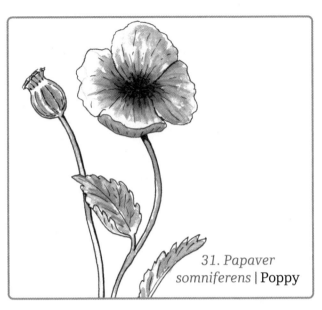

31. Papaver somniferens | Poppy

31.

Papaver somniferens | Poppy

Poppy is cold and dry and, there are three types of it, the flower of one is white, of another it is red as is the rose, of the third, red and pale; and this is less effective than the other two. This is known as the wild poppy. But of all, the best has the white flower.

Of the tender seed heads men make opium: they cut a little the outer skin of the poppy seed head, and the latex that comes out of it they take and save it until it is dry and this opium is good for many medicines. Some other men take the seed heads as they grow with her latex and they grind it and squeeze out of it the juice and dry it in the sun. This is not so effective as is the first method.

The first is called opium, and the second is called *capitellum*; the white flower of the poppy is called *miconium*.

PRIMARILY

For sleep ~
The poppy that has rose coloured flowers - this seed when it is pressed produces an oil. This oil has a very good flavour and will make you sleep well.

A decoction of any of these poppies made into a warm drink will give a sick person a good sleep, but if the patient is likely to die soon, this will happen if the sick person's face is washed with this liquid.

Apply this ointment (opium mixed with oil of roses, saffron and woman's milk) under the ears and it will make you sleep, it is absorbed through the skin, a smaller amount is required when used in this way than when taken orally.

For coughs ~
The seed drunk as a tea helps you sleep well, and it stops the debilitating cough. But, be careful that you don't drink or eat more than a penny weight of the seeds at the most, because anyone who takes more than this, shall often die or at the least fall into a deep sleep.

For cheeks that are swollen ~
A plaster of poppy leaves will reduce the swellings of the cheeks.

For Holy Fire/ergot poisoning ~
This plaster will heal the sickness that is known as the Holy Fire and in Latin *sacer ignis*.

For the voice ~
If the voice becomes sharp or hard, or is cold or after singing or drinking or over eating, apply this medicine to the throat as a poultice, and it will make the voice soft and light.

It is said that Greeks call all types of poppy *miconium*. The white poppy is far nobler and better than the other two. When the seed heads of this poppy are full of latex, gather and warm in two parts water and the third honey until all this together has the consistency of fine honey, and, keep this decoction, because it is healing for many illnesses. This decoction eaten or drunk will make you sleep well.

For coughs ~
This decoction will heal the cough, cause constipation and dry up mucous that comes down the back of the throat.

For headaches ~
As I have mentioned before, the opium made of the tender seed heads of this poppy, if you mix it with it oil of roses and apply to the head, this ointment will ease headaches and enable you to sleep easily.

For the ear ~
If you add sweet smelling saffron stigmas to this mixture and hold this mixture in the ear it will ease earache.

For hot gout of the foot ~
Blend this ointment with woman's milk and saffron, and this mixture when applied frequently will heal the hot gout.

Side effects ~
The black seed drunk with wine will make you costive/constipated.

It will ease a women's heavy periods.

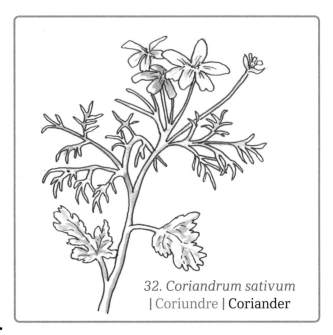

32. Coriandrum sativum
| Coriundre | Coriander

32.

Coriandrum sativum | Coriundre | Coriander

Coriander is cold.

Galen said that coriander has a somewhat stern and stiff quality because it will kill worms found in the womb and the discomfort of the stomach due to worms - drink coriander with wine or vinegar mixed together.

PRIMARILY

For the testicles ~
Coriander blended with raisons and honey and applied as a plaster will reduce swellings of the testicles.

For the flux (diarrhoea) ~
Coriander seed drunk frequently with water will stop diarrhoea.

For Holy Fire (ergot poisoning) ~
Take white lead and the 'froth'of silver (this is a by- product of the process of separating silver from lead), mix them together and grind them until they are very small, then add to this mixture the juice of coriander and vinegar; to these 4 mix oil of roses and grind all this together. This precious ointment will ease the pain of Holy Fire and ease the hot swellings associated with it. If all this seems too expensive then using coriander juice with fine vinegar will give some relief.

For excessive heat ~

The juice of coriander mixed with crumbs of white clean bread will cool all types of excessive heat.

The juice mixed with bean meal will heal wenns or ulcers and infected welks.

Many men have written that the corns of coriander seeds eaten before the tertian fever has begun to cause trembling of the limbs will prevent the fever from developing.

And the seed will have the same effect if it is gathered in the morning before the sun has risen and then put it under the patient's head.

Xenocrates said that if a woman's period should fail to arrive, up to five days after it was due she should eat coriander seed corns to bring on her period.

Some men warn that the custom of eating coriander will bring on an early death or some other great mischief.

Anyone who prefers not to eat pepper due to its great heat in sauces and food can use coriander instead because it is cold and it will cool the heat of pepper.

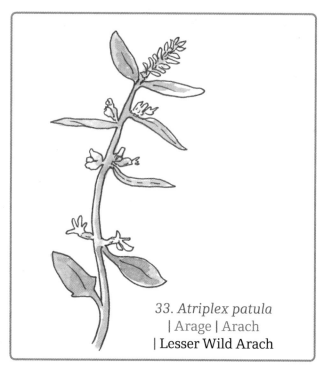

33. *Atriplex patula*
| Arage | Arach
| Lesser Wild Arach

33. *Atriplex patula* | Arage | Arach | Lesser Wild Arach

Arach is cold in the first degree and moist in the second.

PRIMARILY

For hardness ~
Arach when eaten has a laxative effect.

A plaster of arach soaked or fresh will ease various swellings and draw out nails.

This plaster will draw out nails, or spears and the sting of the hornet and it also heals Holy Fire.

For gout ~
Arach ground up small with nitrum, honey and vinegar will ease gout.

For jaundice ~
Galen said an infusion of arach seed drunk frequently will ease and heal jaundice.

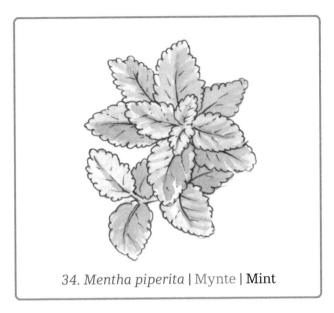

34. Mentha piperita | Mynte | **Mint**

34.

Mentha piperita | **Mynte** | **Mint**

Mint is hot and dry in the second degree

PRIMARILY

For the stomach and worms ~

Mint drunk as a tea helps the digestion, comforts the stomach, stops vomiting and kills worms in the belly.

Wash the testicles with the water that mint is soaked in and it will heal various pains and discomfort in that area.

Warmed mint juice taken as a drink will clarify the voice.

For breasts ~

Mint ground up and applied to the breasts will increase milk production in the nursing mother.

For the ear ~

Hold in the ear the juice of mint blended with honey, this will ease earache.

For the tongue ~

Rub the tongue often with mint and it will heal the rawness of the tongue.

Mint juice mixed with sapa (new wine boiled to a syrup), given at sunrise to a pregnant woman will ease morning sickness.

For dog bites ~
Mint ground up with salt and applied to the bite will heal it.

For him that spits blood/haemoptysis ~
The juice of mint mixed with vinegar helps anyone who spits blood.

Mint juice placed into the space in front of the cervix ensures that the woman shall not conceive at that time.

Mint juice dries ulcers/tumours.

Mint ground up and applied to the head will heal wounds of the head.

Mint juice mixed with whey will not allow cheese to rot. Lay the green mint about the cheese and it will act as a preservative.

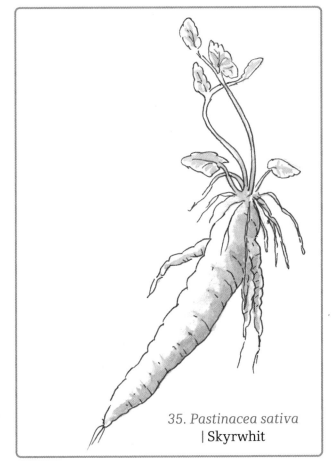

35. *Pastinacea sativa*
| Skyrwhit

35.
Pastinacea sativa
| Skyrwhit

The only parts of skyrwhit that have value are the seeds and the root.

'Who so ever eats a lot of skyrwhit will be very lustful.'

PRIMARILY

For the spleen, the liver and the loins ~
A decoction of the roots in mulsa will heal the illnesses of the spleen and of the liver and the ache of the loins .

For the chincough ~
These roots soaked in milk and made into a decoction will help ease the chronic cough and also stops diarrhoea.

For the testicles ~
Some men say that if you hang pieces of this root about the neck it will ease the swelling of the testicles.

For serpents ~

It is said that if you carry some skyrwhit about your person or eat some root it will protect you from snake bites.

For toothache ~

Rub the teeth and gums with some skyrwhit root and it will ease toothache.

For scorpion stings ~

If you are stung by a scorpion drink a decoction of skyrwhit seed to alleviate the pain.

In the same way it will reduce the swelling of a woman's womb if it is due to a false pregnancy.

For cancers ~

This seed ground up small with honey and laid over the cancer will help the sufferer feel more comfortable.

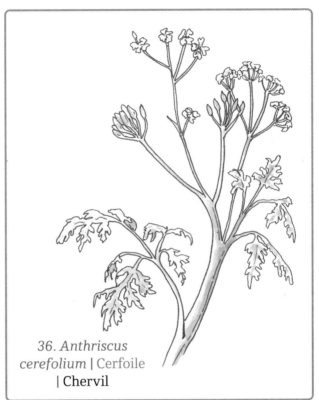

36. *Anthriscus cerefolium* | Cerfoile | Chervil

36. *Anthriscus cerefolium* | Cerfoile | Chervil

Chervil is hot and sharp.

PRIMARILY

For cancers ~
Chervil ground up with honey and laid over a cancer will help heal it.

For the side ~
Chervil drunk with wine will help ease the ache of the side if you bind the herb to the side that aches.

For the slimy exudates ~
Chervil drunk with mulsa will dry up the slime.

For cold ~
Massage the body with oil that has had chervil soaked in it to heal a cold.

For griping of the intestines due to worms ~

Drink chervil dissolved in strong vinegar to kill the worms of the stomach and the intestines.

Chervil drunk with wine will encourage urination and bring on a women's periods.

For swellings ~

A plaster of chervil, old pig fat and of new wax mixed together will heal not only the parotids (salivary glands) that swell in the face but all manner of swellings as long as it is applied regularly.

For vomiting ~

Chervil mixed with fine vinegar will stop diarrhoea and vomiting.

For the opening of the groin ~

Apply a poultice of chervil to the cervix and drink the juice of chervil to open up the groin area if it has narrowed.

For the head ~

Specific for vertigo, boil the herb and bind it to the temples and the front of the head, but, first wash the head in the water that the chervil has been boiled in and this will heal the sickness.

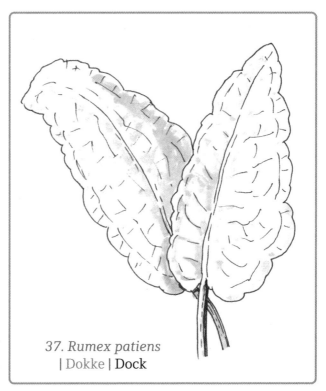

37. Rumex patiens
| Dokke | Dock

37.
Rumex patiens
| Dokke
| Dock

The dock is called paradilla and lapacium as well. There are four types of dock and all have equal value in medicine.

All the docks are hot, stiff and stern in virtue.

PRIMARILY

For the stomach ~
Drink dock juice to comfort the stomach, it brings on belching which releases wind trapped in the stomach.

For the scab ~
The water that the dock is soaked in will soothe the 'biting' itch and the scab that tears the skin (*scabies?*), bathe and wash the area frequently.

The roots of dock soaked in wine and applied to the area will heal the enlarged glands and pustules that erupt during fevers.

For toothache ~
A decoction of docks rolled about in the mouth will heal toothache and the swollen uvula.

If you hang dock roots about your neck you will not suffer from morbid swellings or fever .

For bloody dysentery ~

Drinking this decoction will help heal the bloody dysentery and diseases of the thighs.

For the ears ~

This warm decoction dropped into the ear will heal earache.

For the spleen ~

Dock roots soaked in strong vinegar, ground up and applied to the area of the swollen spleen will help reduce it even though the swelling is severe, and this will dry up the humours that annoy the spleen.

The wine or water that dock roots have been soaked in, when drunk, will stop a woman's period and eliminate gall stones, this will heal jaundice.

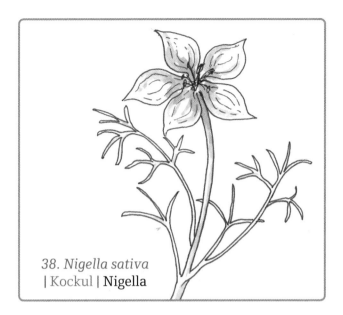

38. Nigella sativa
| Kockul | **Nigella**

38.

Nigella sativa
| Kockul
| **Nigella**

Kockul is known in
Greek lolium and in
Latin nigella.

PRMARILY

For cancers ~
Nigella ground up with raisins and bryony and a little salt make
this mixture into a plaster, lay this on the cancer and this will
cleanse it. This plaster will also cure irritated and eating wounds
- scab or leprosy that is known as zerna.

For the scab or leper ~
This leprosy is like the scab that is called serpigo. It helps also
other types of leprosy.

Nigella, brimstone and excrement and lily seed, grind all this
together with wine and soak in wine to make a plaster and this
will heal the previously mentioned sicknesses, as will an
ointment made of the same ingredients.

For deep seated abscesses ~
This ointment will in the same way reduce kernells. And break
up and soften deep seated abscesses and swellings.

For sciatic pain ~
A plaster of nigella soaked in mulsa and ground
up small with frankincense and saffron will
heal sciatic pain.

A drink of nigella given to a woman in labour
will help speed up the delivery of the child.

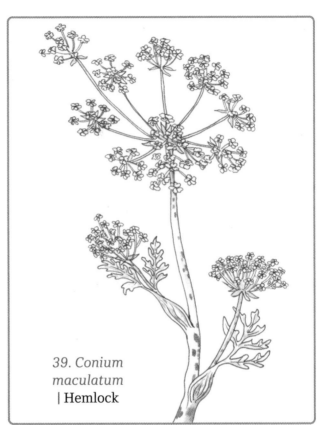

39. Conium maculatum | Hemlock

39.
Conium maculatum | **Hemlock**

Kind, cold and deadly

PRIMARILY

Hemlock kills in the manner of cold venom, and whoever is poisoned with hemlock their skin becomes spotty, people think that this is a sign that proves the source of the poison which caused the death. This drink was used at one time as a way of committing suicide by people that were condemned to death at Athens. The Greek Socrates died by drinking hemlock. How you make this poison is not for me to tell, there is nothing written here that will cause harm, but only that which should heal and help people. If anybody is poisoned with hemlock, drink strong warm wine, and this should prevent death. But although this herb is perilous as a drink it is good for plasters and other medicines.

For the eyes ~

Anoint the sore eyes with the juice of hemlock all around them, and this will have a cooling effect. Or grind green hemlock leaves and apply them to the face, this will have the same effect.

Holy Fire/ergot poisoning ~

This poultice will heal Holy Fire and the sore that is called herpes.

For breasts ~

Amasilaus says that if a maid anoints her breasts with hemlock juice when they begin to swell, they will remain small.

The green hemlock ground up and bound to the breasts dries up breast milk.

A plaster of hemlock applied frequently to the penis reduces lechery and also the flux of the seed.

For gout ~

A plaster of hemlock melded with the froth of silver/litharge of silver and pig fat is very effective in cooling the hot gout, the herb is also effective used on its own.

For harmful heat ~

Hemlock ground and applied to the area is good for cooling harmful heat.

(Interestingly there is no mention in Macer of using hemlock in mixtures to produce a deep sleep similar to that produced by general anaesthetics, although it has been found in the drains at Soutra in combination with opium and henbane, the other two main ingredients of a mixture which is known to have this effect).

40. Mentha pulegium
Pyloile | Brother Wort | **Pennyroyal**

40.
Mentha pulegium | Pyloile | Brother Wort | Pennyroyal

Hot and dry in the 3rd degree

PRIMARILY

If a woman is with child and drinks this herb frequently she will abort her child, if this herb is ground up small and drunk in mulsa/wine it will put out a warpling from the womb

Pennyroyal drunk in warm wine brings on women's periods and also delivers women of the after-birth. The after-birth of women is called in Latin *secunda* or *secundina*. This name is strange to many folks, so, I will explain what is meant by this name.

A child that is not come forth has the 'egg shell' going about him and is covered all over with a thin skin that is made of his mothers seed, the child breaks the skin as he is born – as a chick breaks the egg shell when it comes forth. This skin is called secunda or secundina. When the child is out of the mother's womb his skin comes out afterwards. And if the skin stays behind in the mother's womb after the child is born longer than it should death may follow in the mother or else some other great sickness. (*Retained afterbirth*)

For the limbs ~
Grind pennyroyal finely with salt and honey and mead - this ointment will help the limbs that have been drawn together and shortened, if it is applied often. *(Possibly due to tendons that have become 'shortened' due to injury).*

For phlegm ~
Powder of pennyroyal eaten with honey or drunk will dissolve and thin viscose phlegm.

For the breast ~
Pennyroyal eaten on an empty stomach or if pulped and drunk will heal all illnesses of the heart and breast.

For the stomach ~
Pennyroyal eaten or drunk with pusca or with diluted vinegar will cure pains in the stomach.

For venom ~
Pennyroyal drunk with wine will heal the venomous bites of adders.

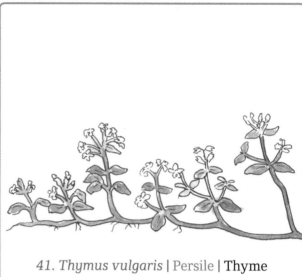

41. Thymus vulgaris | Persile | Thyme

41.
Thymus vulgaris | Persile | Thyme

Persile is known as serpillum in Latin because it creeps forth like a serpent.

Thyme is hot and dry.

PRIMARILY

For the head ache ~
Grind thyme with vinegar and oil of roses and with this ointment rub onto the front of the head and this will ease headaches.

For venomous beasts ~
The smoke of thyme drives away all serpents and all other beasts that cast venom out of their mouths, and because of this it is the tradition of reapers to mix thyme in with their meat, so that all venomous beasts will flee from them and do no harm, if it so happens that they fall asleep when weary.

For bites ~
Thyme drunk as an infusion heals poisonous bites and also if it is applied to the area in the form of a plaster.

Thyme increases urination and relives the griping of the belly.

For the spleen ~
Thyme drunk often with vinegar will help the spleen.

For him that spits blood ~
Thyme drunk with honey helps soothe and heal people who spit blood.

For the liver ~
Thyme drunk with wine will ease the ache of the liver and bring on a woman's period.

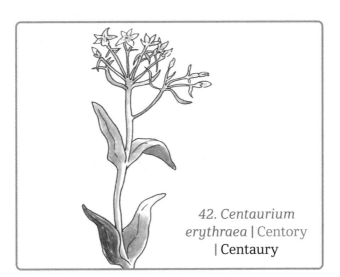

42. *Centaurium erythraea* | Centory | Centaury

42.

Centaurium erythraea | Centory | Centaury

There are two types of centaury the greater and the lesser, the greater is virtually unknown by most people and so I will concentrate on the lesser/smaller and talk about its virtues.

This lesser centaury is drying and is known as a febrifuge - and is cooling.

PRIMARILY

For wounds ~

The lesser centaury will heal new wounds and a plaster of it will reduce the scarring of old wounds.

For sciatica ~

A decoction of centaury given as an enema will help ease the pain of sciatica significantly.

For wounds ~

This herb drunk with wine helps heal wounds wonderfully.

To staunch /stop bleeding ~

Centaury stops a wound from bleeding and if you bathe in a decoction of it, it quickly eases the pain of the wound.

For sinews ~

This decoction will help ease sore ligaments in a similar way.

The juice of centaury when it is drunk will bring on a women's period and cause the delivery of a warpling/deformed child if there is one.

For venom ~

It is said that centaury drunk with wine will neutralise venom.

For the eyes ~

Centaury blended with honey will cleanse the duskiness of the eye (cataracts).

Take the juice of centaury at harvest time and dry it in the sun and keep it safe because it will heal all the illnesses that have been mentioned and it's good for you.

43. Teucrium chamaedrys | Gamodreos | Germander

43.
Teucrium chamaedrys | Gamodreos | Germander

Gamodreos in Greek is called *gamandrea* in Latin.

It is a hot herb and dry in the third degree.

PRIMARILY

This herb drunk in water will deliver a woman of a child that is dead in her womb and also it will heal coughs.

For bruises ~
It is good for bruises if it is drunk blended with vinegar.

For the spleen and dropsy/heart failure ~
This herb drunk with wine dries the spleen and brings on a woman's period. In the early stages it will also heal the dropsy/heart failure that is cold.

For venomous bites ~
It will heal deadly venomous bites.

To all conditions that have already been mentioned this herb will help if it is ground up and placed onto the affected area.

For wounds ~
This herb ground up and mixed with honey and applied to the area will cleanse a wound even if it is old.

For the eyes ~
An ointment made from the juice of this herb and honey makes the eyes bright and clears away cataracts if it is used often.

For cold ~
Mix the ground herb with oil and massage the body, this will have a warming effect.

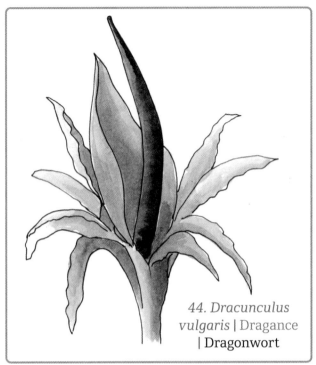

44. Dracunculus vulgaris | Dragance | Dragonwort

44. *Dracunculus vulgaris* | Dragance | Dragonwort

Dragance or adderstongue is spotted like a snake.

PRIMARILY

For venom ~
If you cover yourself with the juice of this herb you will not be bitten by an adder or any other venomous snake.

Dragonwort drunk with wine will heal adder bites.

For the ear ~
The juice of dragonwort seed mixed with oil and held in the ear will heal earache.

For polyps ~
Dip wool into the juice of this plant and place it in the nose this will heal nasal polyps.

For cancer ~
In the same way it is a great help to cancers.

For the eyes ~
With the juice of dragonwort roots you can heal cataracts and many other diseases that affect the eyes - if you apply this juice to the eyes or the juice mixed with honey.

It is said that 13 *corns* of dragonwort seeds drunk with pusca/wine will clear cataracts.

If a woman that is with child smells the fragrance of dragonwort flowers when the flower is withered she will be delivered of a warpling and the same thing will happen if the root of dragonwort is placed onto her cervix.

For catarrh ~
The powder of dragonwort roots mixed with honey will heal coughs and dry up catarrh if it is eaten frequently.

For the breast ~
This same is a great help to those who spit blood and it also cures afflictions of the breast permanently.

Dragonwort is good roasted and eaten and also valuable as a decoction.

For wounds ~
Dragonwort roots drunk with wine cause lechery, increase urination and clean foul wounds and cure fistulas and heal wounds.

For spots ~
Dragonwort with vinegar heals spots.

For chilblains ~
The water that dragonwort roots have been soaked in will heal chilblains particularly those found on the heel, they occur due to poor circulation in cold weather and are commonly called mula.

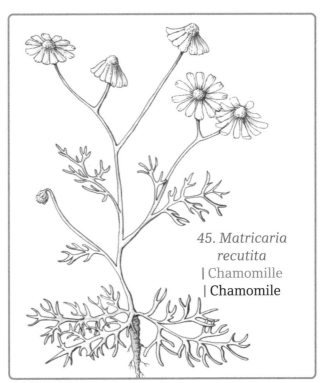

45. *Matricaria recutita*
| Chamomille
| Chamomile

45.
Matricaria recutita
| Chamomille
| Chamomile

All are hot and dry in the first degree.

Asclepius praised hugely chamomylle; this is known as chamomile. This herb is sweet in flavour and short in substance. It is very similar to a herb that is known as amarisca, because it has a strong fragrance and has a bitter taste. So alike are these herbs that when you see them together the only way to tell them apart is by their taste. Authors say that there are three types of chamomile, and the only way to distinguish one from another is by the colour of their flowers.

All have a yellow disc florets in the middle, but each species of these three has beside this flower petals of various colours which surround the yellow disc florets in the centre - these are white, black or purple. Anthemis has ray florets standing around the yellow which are purple in colour, this is the strongest. The second is known as lenchantemon/white ox-eye daisy, and this has white petals around the yellow. The third is known as crisantemon /chrysanthemum and has black flowers around the yellow.

PRIMARILY

For the stone ~

Any of these drunk frequently with wine stimulate urination and dissolve bladder stones; and bring on a woman's periods, it is equally effective if the herb is infused in a bath and the woman bathes in the infusion.

For the stomach ~

It stops the stirring and swelling of the stomach.

This infusion might help to get rid of spots or freckles on the skin.

Finely ground up chamomile mixed with honey and applied externally will have a similar effect.

For jaundice ~

A decoction of this herb when drunk eases jaundice and help heal diseases of the liver.

Chamomile drunk with wine will deliver a woman of her dead child.

For the fever ~

Infuse chamomile in oil and rub on to anyone who has a fever. This ointment will have a warming effect and ease the symptoms of the fever.

This ointment drives away the evil that swells the flanks.

If you drink a dragme weight of Chamomile with wine this will neutralise poisonous bites.

For the spleen ~

Plinius said that whoever drinks two dragme weight each day of chamomile for 40 days with two ciatus of good clean white wine, this will have a cleansing effect on the spleen, particularly if the area is washed with the mixture as well.

For the leper ~

This chamomile chewed and applied to the area will heal all types of leprosy particularly the one that causes an ulcer or fistula in the inner angle of the eye; and it also cleans septic wounds.

For the head ~

Chamomile is known to ease headaches that are due to the heat of fever.

Often in the head deep seated abscesses or swellings develop, these are swellings the Greeks call 'eruptions' or 'rash'. Take green chamomile and infuse it in oil, and if you do not have any green, use the dry herb and soak it in vinegar and cover the head all over with this mixture, there is no ointment that helps heal this condition more effectively.

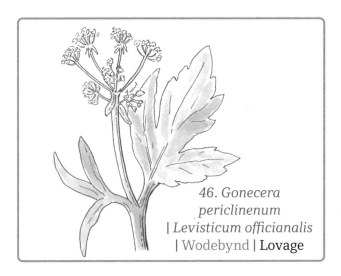

46. *Gonecera periclinenum*
| *Levisticum officianalis*
| Wodebynd | Lovage

46.

Gonecera periclinenum | Levisticum officianalis | Wodebynd | Lovage

Wodebynd is known as *caprifolium* and *ligusticum* - it is called this in the country of Liguri where this herb grows everywhere.

It is hot and dry both in the third degree. The most virtue of this herb is in the root and seed.

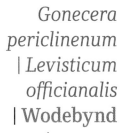

PRIMARILY

For the stomach ~
This herb drunk with wine will reduce the swelling of the stomach, and it also helps digestion.

For entrails/intestines ~
In the same way it helps all the sores of the 'entrails' and the' inner parties'. Also increases urination and brings on a woman's period.

For venomous bites ~
This herb helps against all venomous bites if it is soaked and steeped in wine and then ground small and drunk, a part of this mixture should be applied to the place that has been bitten as well.

For colic pains ~
This herb either eaten or drunk will ease the pain of colic. And not only the seeds but also a decoction of the roots will also have this effect.

Dangerous for eyesight ~
The seed of this herb helps to improve digestion. Strabus confirms this and also that this herb may harm eyesight if it is taken as a drink or in food and therefore he suggested that the seed should only be used in medicines. But I don't know whether he found this out for himself or got it from other books and authors. This I know well, old men rate this herb very highly. All I know is that Strabus is the only author who mentions that this herb might cause harm.

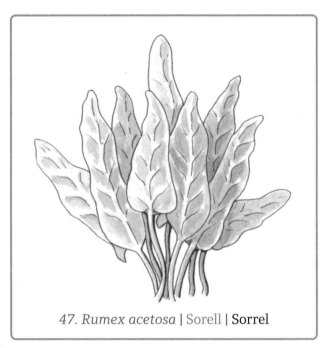

47. *Rumex acetosa* | Sorell | Sorrel

47.
Rumex acetosa | Sorell | Sorrel

This herb is right cold and dry both in the third degree.

PRIMARILY

For Ergot poisoning/Holy Fire ~

A plaster of this herb will ease the pain of Holy Fire and the illness that is called herpeta mordax/ gnawing herpes - This is a very painful eruption, and it will also heal swellings of the eye.

For gout ~

This will heal the swellings that creep over the body and it soothes burns. It is very cooling to the hot gout if the affected area is covered with the green sorrel leaves or if the leaves are bruised and mixed with flour and then placed onto the inflamed area.

For headaches ~

It is said that the juice of sorrel mixed with oil of roses will help ease the chronic headache known as cephalargia.

For diarrhoea ~
Sorrel drunk with wine will stop haemorrhaging from the womb whatever the cause. It also reduces the flow of a woman's period if it is very heavy. If sorrel is bruised and laid onto the cervix it will have the same effect.

For worms in the belly ~
Sorrel drunk with wine will kill round worms in the stomach and also it will save you from all poisons.

Sorrel juice rubbed onto the body cheers you up and makes you happy.

Men say that whoever carries some sorrel, they will not be stung by a scorpion.

For hearing ~
Sorrel juice held in the ear improves hearing and also eases earache, you can use it on its own or you can add oil of roses to the juice.

Sorrel eaten frequently will help people who spit blood.

The flavour is as tart as vinegar and it is found growing in gravelly meadows and beside water.

Many men have eaten this herb in times past and they have reported that it is very effective in healing many illnesses.

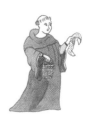

For a visual experience of uprooting the mandrake please flick through the pages of this book and watch the monk carefully...

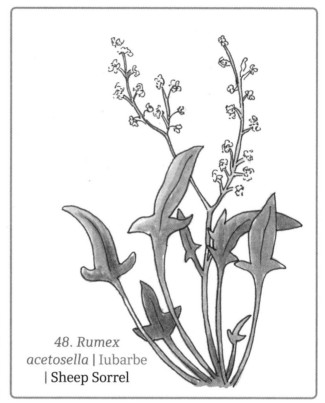

48. *Rumex acetosella* | Iubarbe | Sheep Sorrel

48.
Rumex acetosella | Iubarbe | Sheep Sorrel

Iubarb is a type of sorrel when it is green and fresh it is called senegrene. This is the lesser sorrel.

Plinius said that this is like the previous sorrel and that this is as good and useful to all the conditions already mentioned.

PRIMARILY

For the eyes ~
In the morning sometimes eyelids are glued shut with a type of phlegm or exudate, the juice of this herb applied around the eyelids dissolves this phlegm very effectively.

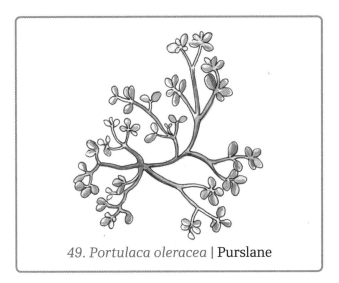

49. Portulaca oleracea | Purslane

49.

Portulaca oleracea | Purslane

Purslane is commonly called foal-foot and in Greek adragmis.

This is cold in the second degree and moist in the third degree.

PRIMARILY

For fevers and the stomach ~
This is good for the type of fever called 'burning fever'. Also to the stomach, particularly if the herb is bruised and laid onto the stomach.

In the same way the juice of this herb is soothing when it is drunk.

For heat ~
Eat this herb as a green vegetable and it will have a cooling effect.

For the flux/diarrhoea ~
This herb either eaten or drunk will ease the flow of the flux of blood out of the womb.

This herb will ease toothache.

For the eyes ~
For eyes that are swollen bruise this herb and apply it onto the eyes.

For womb ~
This herb when eaten will not allow the heat of the sun to harm you. Also when you eat this herb with salt and wine it relaxes the womb.

For the bladder ~
This herb when eaten will ease the ache of the bladder (cystitis), and it helps people who spit blood. Plinius said that sour dock that is sorrel has almost the same virtues as this herb.

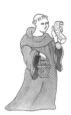

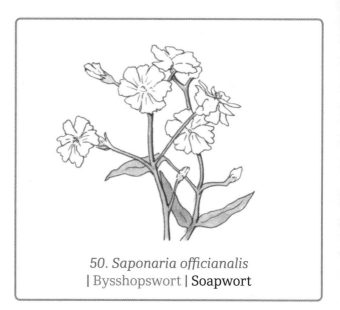

50. Saponaria officianalis
| Bysshopswort | **Soapwort**

50.
Saponaria officianalis
| Bysshops-wort
| Soapwort

Bysshopeswort is called structon or ostructon.

This is hot and dry

PRIMARILY

For the liver ~
The root of this herb ground up and drunk with wine will ease all sicknesses of the liver and the swellings of the spleen and heal jaundice.

For the stone ~
In the same way it softens the hardness that is known as cirrhosis and dissolves stones in the bladder allowing them to be flushed away and also it brings on women's periods.

For the cough ~
In the same way it eases the flow of urine which heals the cough.

For haemoptysis ~
This is very healing for people who spit blood if it is drunk regularly.

This herb will enable a woman to give birth to a dead child if it is put around the cervix. Also it will bring on a woman's period if it is late.

For the leper ~
The juice of this herb mixed with vinegar and flour will cleanse sores if it is applied to them.

For welks/sores ~
A plaster of the juice of this herb mixed thoroughly with barley flour will heal the welk.

For the scab ~
This herb combined with vinegar and flour and the juice of scabious and rubbed on to the scab will heal it.

For the head ~
The juice of this herb mixed with honey and blended well together eases the humours of the head if it is inhaled through the nose.

To aid sneezing ~
The powder of this herb drawn in through the nose with the juice of white hellebore will make you sneeze, violently.

For jaundice ~
This same powder mixed with woman's milk and drawn in through the nose will help anyone who has jaundice.

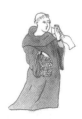

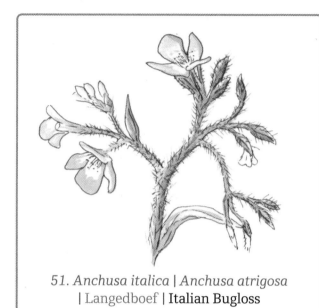

51. Anchusa italica | Anchusa atrigosa
| Langedboef | Italian Bugloss

51.
Anchusa italica | Anchusa atrigosa | Langedboef | Italian Bugloss

Langedboe, is known as ox tongue. It is excellent at cooling the burnt red colour associated with great heat and high blood pressure, if it is drunk regularly with wine.

PRIMARILY

For colour ~
It will heal anyone who has a heart condition.

For the lungs ~
This herb drunk frequently will eliminate all the wicked humours of the lungs.

For the pain of sciatica ~
The juice of this herb drunk frequently in warm water will ease the pain of sciatica.

Wise men say that drinking the wine that this herb is soaked in will help improve your memory.

A decoction of this herb has a cheering, up lifting effect when it is taken as a drink.

For the tertian fever ~
Make a decoction of roots and seeds of this herb and drink it frequently to ease/cool the tertian fever.

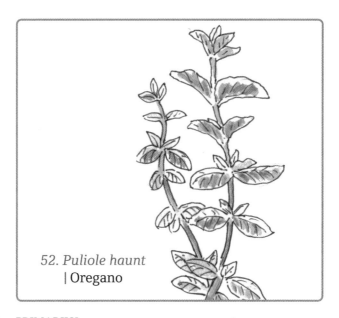

52. Puliole haunt
| Oregano

52.
Puliole haunt
| Oregano

Puliole haunt is known in Latin as oreganum. This is hot and dry in the third degree.

PRIMARILY

For bites ~
A decoction of this herb drunk regularly in wine will cure all poisonous bites.

For poisons ~
This decoction drunk in mulsa will protect anyone who has drunk the poison aconite and in the same way it is protection against many other poisons.

For bruises ~
This herb is good for bruises if it is eaten and drunk frequently.

For dropsy (heart failure) ~
This herb supports the heart and dries up the swellings associated with heart failure.

For black cholera ~
This herb drunk in mulsa will heal the black cholera

A drink of this herb or a decoction of it or a poultice will bring on a woman's period.

For coughs ~
The powder of this herb eaten with honey will heal coughs.

For jaundice ~
Frequent bathing in a decoction of this herb will get rid of itching and spots on the skin and jaundice as well.

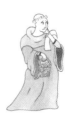

For the cheeks ~
The juice of this green herb when drunk will help reduce swellings of the cheeks and the uvula.

For the mouth ~
The juice held in the mouth and rolled often about will heal blisters of the mouth.

For the head ~
This juice combined with oil of iris held in at the nose will allow the blood to run out that might otherwise harm the head.

For the ear ~
The juice of oregano mixed with a little woman's milk held in the ear will ease earache.

To slay noxious beasts ~
This juice mixed with onions and roses, put it in the sun for 15 days in a brass pot, over this time it will dry up and drive away all dangerous beasts if it is put under the bed.

For the stomach ~
This juice drunk with good white wine will help gluttons that have eaten so much that their stomach can't digest the food.

This juice drunk with hot water will ease any discomfort of the stomach.

For the bruise, scab and scalding ~
Take some dry wool and soak it in oregano juice mixed with oil and vinegar, lay this over any bruise, scab or scalding and it will heal it.

For worms in the stomach ~
Drink a decoction of this herb to eliminate worms from the stomach.

For the teeth ~
This herb eases toothache.

The juice of this herb drunk frequently helps all areas within the body.

To encourage sweating ~
Drink the juice mixed with a fig ground up very small and this will open the pores and make the sweat run out.

For the thighs ~
A plaster made of the juice of oregano mixed with wheat meal and laid to the place that aches will ease the discomfort.

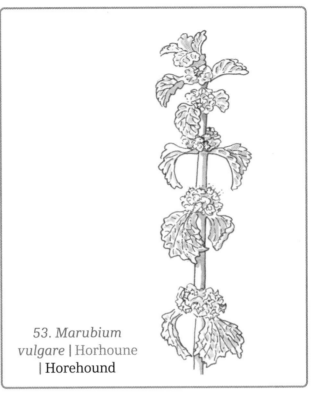

53. *Marubium vulgare* | Horhoune | Horehound

53.
Marubium vulgare | Horhoune | Horehound

Horhoune is called in Latin marubium and in Greek prassion.

It is hot and dry both in the second degree.

PRIMARILY

For coughs ~
A decoction of the whole herb or just of the seed will help soothe coughs very effectively.

For the breast ~
This drink will heal many sicknesses of the breast and it works even more effectively if iris is mixed with it.

For the chink (chincough) ~
This herb drunk in old wine will neutralise all poison and help ease the 'chink' and the common cough.

For women suffering an extended labour ~
It will shorten a women's labour if it is drunk during labour, it also speeds up the release of the afterbirth.

For wounds ~
This herb mixed with honey will cleanse wounds and heal bruises that have broken the skin.

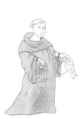

For the sides ~
It is said that this decoction will ease the ache of the sides.

You can use the fresh juice or dry the juice so that it can be kept over winter - it still works just as effectively

For the fever and the catarrh ~
This juice drunk in water will eliminate fever and catarrh.

For the eyes ~
This juice mixed with wine or with honey will help improve eye sight.

For jaundice ~
The juice breathed in through the nose will help anyone who suffers from jaundice.

Men say that the juice combined with rose oil dripped into the ear will ease earache.

For worms in the belly ~
Warm horehound and wormwood in wine and bind them to the navel, this will kill the worms in the belly.

Men say that is not good to eat or drink horehound if you have bladder or kidney disease.

If you want to 'dodge the imp' [sic] of horehound after taking it eat some fennel seed and this will protect you.

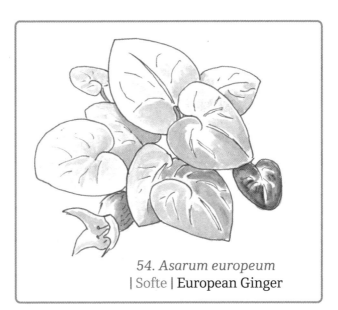

54. *Asarum europeum*
| Softe | European Ginger

54.

Asarum europeum | Softe | European Ginger

A softe or moleyn is called asarum in Greek and in Latin *ulgago*.

This is both hot and dry in the third degree.

PRIMARILY

For the liver ~
When this herb is drunk it stimulates urination and brings on women's periods and helps with all the illnesses of the liver.

For the dropsy/heart failure ~
This herb drunk regularly will help with heart failure and the pain of sciatica.

A decoction of this herb helps heal the sicknesses and sores of the vagina.

For jaundice ~
It is said that drinking a decoction made from this herb will heal jaundice.

As a purgative ~
A decoction of this herb acts as a purgative, cleansing the bowels in a way similar to hellebore but the purging caused by Softe is not as violent as that of hellebore. Do not dread using this purgative as long as you use it according to these guidelines.

When you are going to use this purgative look at the age and the strength of the person that is going to take it, also take the time of year into consideration and whether it is hot or cold or warm. You should only use a little of this herb with children or the old and feeble. If he is of middle age you should use more than the

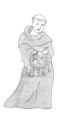

previously mentioned people can tolerate. To him that is fat and strong you use more than when treating someone who is lean and feeble regardless of their age. In a cold time you need to use more than during a hot time of year or location. If the person is used to doing hard physical labour you need to use more than if the person is used to rest and idleness.

If you follow these guidelines you can be confident not only in using this herb but also all the other herbs that purge either by vomiting or through the stomach or womb. Now I have said generally how you should use all manner of herbs but now I will say exactly how you should use this herb.

You should take 30 fresh leaves of this herb and place them in as much wine as you can hold in your mouth and let them infuse over night in the wine. In the morning take out the leaves from the wine and grind them up very small and then put them back into the wine that they were soaked in overnight. Then you should give the sick person the herb softe, that has had fat pork soaked in it and let him drink as much strong white wine as he wants and strain through a cloth the juice of the herb that has been soaking overnight and let him drink this as well. This number of leaves is I know sufficient for a fat and strong man, for others who are not so strong you need to use less of this medicine as I have already mentioned.

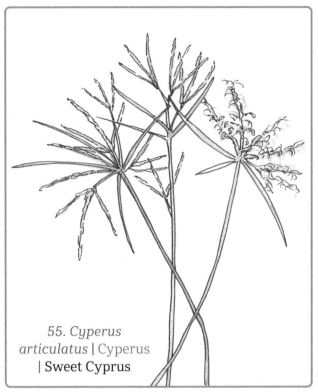

55. Cyperus articulatus | Cyperus | Sweet Cyprus

55.
Cyperus articulatus | Cyperus | Sweet Cyprus

Physicians say that this herb is called *Cyperus* in Latin.

It is hot and dry in the second degree.

PRIMARILY

For urine ~
A drink of this herb acts as a purge and a laxative also opening the flow of urine.

A decoction of this herb will put out of a woman's belly a dead child, if a woman bathes and washes with this decoction.

For the spleen ~
The smoke from this herb will ease the spleen if it is inhaled through the mouth.

If a healthy man makes a tea of this herb it will make him calm and lift his spirits as well.

For the armpits ~
The juice of this herb mixed with oil will ease the inflamed swellings and sores of the armpit if it is rubbed onto the area.

This juice drunk frequently dries up excessive 'humours' and fluids.

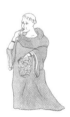

For swellings and wounds ~

The powder of this herb on its own or mixed with honey will clean rotten/septic wounds.

For heart failure ~

This powder is particularly good for inflamed swellings of the mouth if it is taken as a drink and it also comforts the stomach that is feeble and it helps heart failure if it is drunk frequently - by increasing the amount of urine produced thereby reducing water retention - a symptom of heart failure.

For swellings ~

Grind this herb up small and put into strong vinegar and by using this medicine you can heal the creeping swellings.

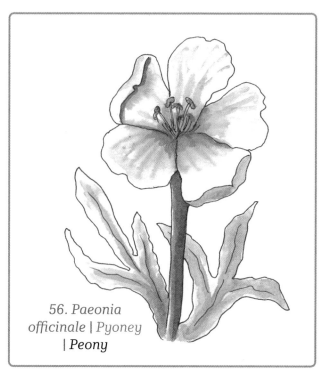

56. *Paeonia officinale* | Pyoney | *Peony*

56.

Paeonia officinale | Pyoney | **Peony**

Pyoney is both hot and dry in the second degree.

PRIMARILY

For the spleen, the liver and the kidneys ~

This tea drunk with well ground almonds and mulsa/wine will help the spleen, the liver and the kidneys.

In the same way it brings on women's periods and eases dysentery.

For the bladder, the head and the stomach ~

A decoction of peony drunk regularly with wine will ease severe aching of the bladder and also it helps soothe headaches that are associated with dizziness accompanied by dimness of sight and stomach ache.

For jaundice ~

This will also help the ache of the sides and jaundice as well.

For dreams ~

Peony seed infusion drunk frequently will help prevent frightening dreams and nightmares .

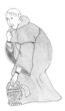

For lunatics ~

Peony boiled and eaten frequently will heal anyone that is considered to be a lunatic.

For epilepsy ~

The root of peony hung about a child's neck that has epilepsy will ease the symptoms according to Galen. Galen tells of a child that had the falling evil at about eight years of age. This child was usually wearing around his neck a peony root. At one point this root fell off, the child instantly fell onto the earth. The root was bound again to his neck and the child was whole again.

Galen had marvelled at this and he took away the root from the child's neck and the child fell down again. And when the root was hung again around the child's neck, the child became whole again, and in this way Galen understood the virtue of this root and of this herb.

Diascorides agrees that this root is good for anyone who has epilepsy if it is drunk frequently or hung about the neck of the patient.

Fifteen red corns of peony seed drunk in wine will stop haemorrhaging from the womb.

The black corns of peony seed are able to heal the various sicknesses of the womb, if the woman patient drinks 15 corns in wine at night just before going to bed.

Peony seed drunk with wine after the birth of a child will cause the woman to deliver the afterbirth/placenta.

There are two types of this herb. The greater is known as the male and the less is called the female. The root of the greater is two palms long and great as a finger. The root of the lesser is divided into many roots

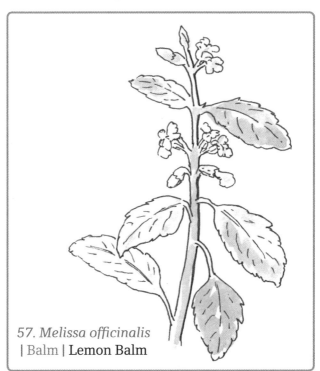

57. *Melissa officinalis*
| Balm | Lemon Balm

57.
Melissa officinalis
| Balm
| Lemon Balm

Among all herbs this is most uplifting, there is no flower that brings as much joy as this herb does.

PRIMARILY

If the beehives are dabbed with the juice of the leaves of this herb, the bees will not fly away and swarm and it is even more effective if there is sweet milk mixed with the juice. The apiarists in olden times kept their swarms by using this method.

Bee or wasp stings ~

This herb ground up and applied to a bee sting will quickly heal the area that has been stung. And in the same way it will heal a wasp sting or a spider bite.

For the breast ~

This herb ground up with salt is used to soothe chronic swellings of the breast and also heals suppurating ulcers.

A woman's ulcerated breasts can be healed by using the juice of this herb soaked in salt, and by taking this drink regularly she is protected against these chronic ulcerations.

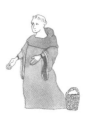

For arthritis ~
A decoction of this green herb drunk frequently will help people who suffer from arthritis and stop the bloody diarrhoea and heal diseases of the womb and it also helps those that have the cough that is known as asthma.

This decoction also cleans wounds and heals sores of the toes.

For bites ~
This herb ground with salt and applied to a dog bite will heal it.

For toothache ~
A decoction of this herb will bring on a woman's period through bathing frequently in it, and it will ease toothache if the decoction is held in the mouth for a while.

For toothache ~
Plinius said that this herb is an excellent remedy for toothache - dig up the herb without using anything made of iron, clean the roots of all the soil and touch the aching tooth with the root three times and after each touch spit and then plant the herb again where it had originally been growing so that the leaves grow as they did before; this Plinius suggested would cure toothache.

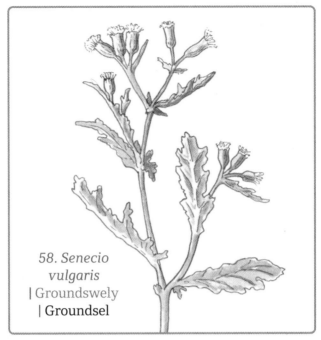

58. *Senecio vulgaris*
| Groundswely
| Groundsel

58.

Senecio vulgaris
| Ground-swely
| Groundsel

Groundeswely we know in Latin *Senecion* and the Greek know her *Yrigenon*. She is known as *Senecion* because her flowers are like horse hairs/grey hairs. This herb grows commonly in walls in gardens.

This herb is cold. the root should not be used in medicines. Gather or use this herb in the morning or at midday.

PRIMARILY

For swellings due to a stroke ~
This herb blended with pig fat and applied to the affected area will reduce swellings that develop as a consequence of having had a stroke.

For the testicles or the ears ~
Grind together the leaves and the flower of this herb, then add to it a little sweet wine and make a plaster and apply it as a hot poultice to the swelling of the ears or of the testicles.

For wounds ~
Add frankincense to this mixture and make a plaster, this plaster will heal sore ligaments and all types of wounds.

For gout ~
This herb ground up finely and mixed with pig fat will heal a wound if it is applied as a plaster, even if it is an old chronic injury; and it will ease the hot gout and all other ailments that effect the legs.

All these ailments will be eased or healed by taking a decoction
of this herb .

Some men say this, do not drink an infusion of this herb because
it will cause a strangled sensation and choking. Plinius, that
great clerk, said that in his experience, some people with
jaundice have drunk this herb with wine and it was very
helpful.

For the bladder ~
Plinius said that this herb drunk with wine will be very helpful
to ailments of the bladder, and he said that many men have
proved this to be so.

For the heart ~
Plinius also said that many men have used this herb within his
knowledge to treat the discomfort and sicknesses of the heart
and of the liver.

For the womb ~
Plinius said also that this herb drunk with vinum passum/raison
wine will reduce the discomfort of the womb and many other
ailments that affect the bowels.

The green herb will be equally effective if it is dipped in vinegar
and eaten.

For the breast ~
This herb is also effective melded with salt and laid to the area
that is affected by an ulcer or swelling or to a large deep seated
abscess of the breast.

For toothache ~
'Here should be some book medicines for the toothache that I
have written at the end of the next chapter before this, and I
wene forsooth that it should be here, but it is myssette for
defaulte of writing.' *(I translate this as: I should have included
this herb when I talked about toothache two chapters ago, but
I forgot to include it, it's my mistake I've put it in the wrong
place).*

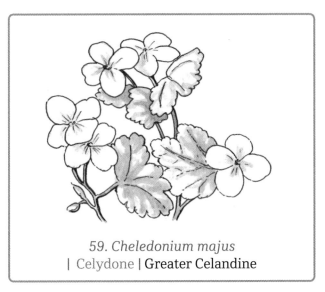

59. Cheledonium majus
| Celydone | Greater Celandine

59.
Cheledonium majus
| Ranunculus ficaria
| Celydone
| **Greater & Lesser Celandine**

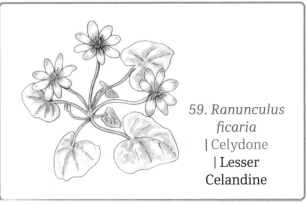

59. Ranunculus ficaria
| Celydone
| Lesser Celandine

Celydone has two types. The first is known by apothecaries, it is the greater and the other is known as the lesser.

PRIMARILY

For the eye ~
Both of them are good for the eyes, Plinius said this and has written,' the swallow makes her chicks able to see with this when they are blind this proves that their eyes are hidden in their heads'.

Men say that this herb flowers when swallows come, and when swallows go away then this herb vanishes and dries up.

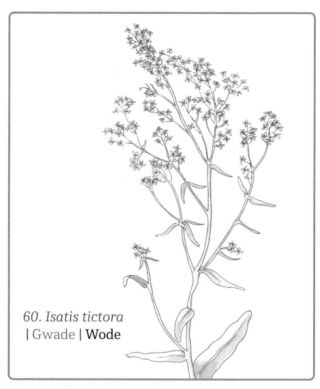

60. Isatis tictora
| Gwade | Wode

60. *Isatis tictora* | Gwade | Wode

Gwade is known in Greek *Ysatis* and in Latyn she is known commonly *Gwasio*.

This herb makes dyers very flatulent.

PRIMARILY

Primarily for adder bites ~
This herb ground up finely and drunk in water helps heal adder bites, make a plaster of this herb and cover the bite with it.

For wounds ~
A plaster made of the leaves of this herb which are ground up into a paste will heal wounds even if they are infected.

Even if a great deal of blood is being lost this herb will stop the bleeding and reduce all types of swellings or tumours.

For freckles ~
Wode heals spots and causes freckles to fade.

Holy Fire ~
Wode will relieve some of the symptoms of Holy Fire/ergot poisoning

For broken bones ~
This herb ground up and mixed with the white of an egg and applied to the fracture will quickly heal broken bones and the pain of the fracture.

Skin ~
And dries and heals the scab that physicians call impetigo.

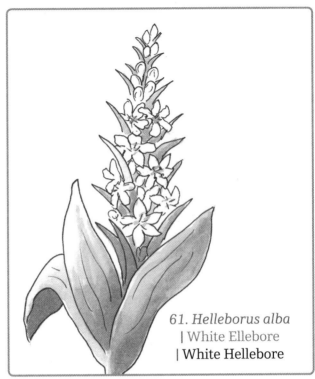

61. *Helleborus alba*
| White Ellebore
| White Hellebore

61. *Helleborus alba* | White Ellebore | White Hellebore

Ellebore has two species. One is white and 'purgeth above' (causes vomiting), that other is black and 'purgeth beneath' (causes violent diarrhoea). It is hot and dry in the third degree. But the white is more violent than the black therefore first will I tell the virtues of the white

PRIMARILY

The white hellebore applied to the cervix in whatever way will deliver a woman of her dead child.

For the head ~

A powder of this herb drawn in at the nose will cause sneezing and in this way will heal sicknesses of the head. Physicians say that if this powder is mixed in with the confections or ointments that have a cleansing affect on the eyes, it is very helpful.

This powder mixed with potage will kill mice.

The same powder mixed with honey will destroy fleas.

For a purgative ~

This powder eaten or drunk will purge by vomiting and this may help ease many severe illnesses, and physicians say it heals old sicknesses and by causing vomiting it heals the disease known as vertigo.

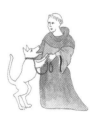

For the falling evil/epilepsy ~

This juice when taken as a drink is helpful to mentally unstable people who are depressed, and helpful for people suffering from epilepsy. It is a very useful in the early stages of heart failure.

For leprosy ~

It cleanses the leper and heals the diseases that are called tetanus and gout.

For the palsy ~

It steadies and stabilises anyone that quakes from the palsy or paralysis. It cures irritations of the womb.

For fevers ~

It is helpful for various sicknesses of the stomach and to sciatica and to old coughs and for fevers - it is better than anything else.

This is medicinal to anyone that has had the ague over many years.

Plinius insists that you should take this herb or its powder only after you have taken seven days to prepare carefully beforehand; eat moist meats and no drink (alcohol) and he is not sure that you should take this herb or her powder as a medicine at all. Plinius also suggests that it should be taken on a merry and hot and clear and bright day, and ensure that it isn't windy.

Plinius says that whoever takes this herb or the powder or juice and doesn't follow this advice will not escape without a serious illness. Plinius says also that this hellebore should be taken infused first in potage or in a type of corn that is known as lentils, and as Plinius says, whoever takes it in this way, it shall do him no harm. Plinius says that this herb shall not be given to young children, neither to old and feeble folks, neither to soft and tender men, neither to him that be soft hearted, nor to lean men, nor to feminine men. Other men should take this herb as a juice in an infusion or in mulsa or baked in bread and in this way it can be taken safely and with benefit. It is said that Philo wrote a book and explained how we should take this hellebore.

And Hippocrates in his teachings mentions this herb. And many
other men have written of the virtues of this herb and taught
how this herb should be taken. And yet I cannot find a clerk that
explains how to take this herb with precise dosages and I have
read a great many books. Therefore I caution that it seems that
they say, it should be taken according to the vigour and age of
the patient. But to me it seems that it is not clearly explained
how to give somebody such a medicine that may bring him into
a sudden peril/death, because of this it is important that the
weight and measure of this herb should be clearly worked out
beforehand but as yet I am not clear on what is a safe dose.
As Plinius has written, Themison used this hellebore in a dose
of two dragmes weight and he said also that the physicians
that followed after him used four dragmes of hellebore. But
nonetheless it seems that he is not clear what weight of the
herb should be taken. But even so he did give some guidelines
to follow - take a dragme or four scruples of the black hellebore
at the most, I surmise therefore that he would suggest that we
should give half the weight of the white hellebore, because it is
much stronger than the black hellebore.

*(I interpret this long and rambling explanation of how or
how not to take hellebore is an interesting piece of writing
effectively saying 'Some great men have used this herb very
effectively, or so it is written but personally I think that it is
very dangerous and I cannot find any clear guidelines on how
to use it. So, if you do use it, it is at your own risk.' And of
course that of your patient).*

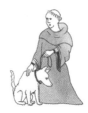

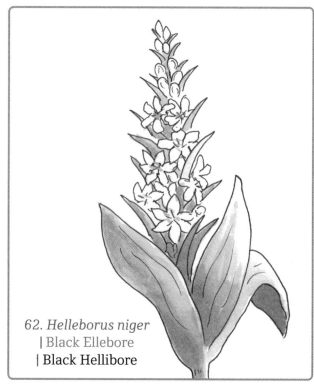

62. *Helleborus niger*
| Black Ellebore
| Black Hellibore

62.
Helleborus Niger
| Black Ellebore
| Black Hellibore

Now the black hellebore is not so violent as the white, neither so much for to dread.

Old men say that the best way to take black hellebore is to cook it with lentils or as mince or hotch-potch, and they say it is medicinal to anyone that is 'wooden' - suffering from tetanus or hemlock poisoning.

PRIMARILY

For the dropsy/heart failure ~
It is good for gout of the foot and to dropsy when fever is present.

For the palsy ~
It helps ease the tremor of palsy, and relieves various sicknesses of the toes and of other joints, if it taken as a drink.

For to soften ~
It drives out through the womb various choleras and phlegm.

For the eyes ~
A decoction of this hellebore when taken as a drink will make eyes clear and bright.

For hardness ~
A plaster of this hellebore will soften a 'hardness' and act as a purgative.

For shingles ~
A twig of this hellebore set in at the neck of the fester known as a fistula, and after two days the twig should be removed.

For the dropsy/heart failure ~
Grind this herb up small and meld with barley meal, and a plaster of this will dry up the accumulated fluids caused by heart failure.

This plaster applied to the cervix will cleanse a woman of her period and bring out the child that is dead in his mother's womb.

For deaf folks ~
This will give hearing to them that are deaf due to sickness, if it is put into the ear and after two days or three taken away.

For lepers ~
A plaster of this hellebore when applied to the area will remove spots and cleanse lepers and heals all scabs.

For toothache ~
The vinegar that this hellebore has been soaked in, held in the mouth a long time, will ease toothache, as men say.

Dosage:
Plinius says use a dragme of black hellebore, and this will move the womb quickly. And Plinius forbids anyone to take or use more than at the most 4 scruples.

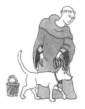

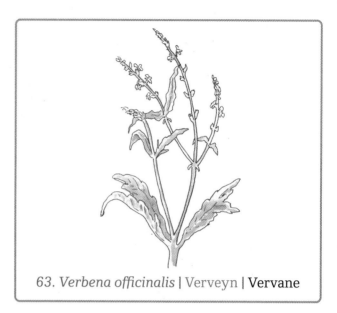

63. Verbena officinalis | Verveyn | **Vervane**

63.

Verbena officinalis | **Verveyn** | **Vervane**

Verveyn known in Greek as *ierobatanum* and *peristerion*. There are two species of verbena and both of them have a very similar effect medicinally.

PRIMARILY

For barking dogs ~
It is said that if you carry verbena in your hand no hound will bark at you where ever you are.

For jaundice ~
Verbena drunk frequently in wine will help heal jaundice.

For bites ~
Verbena blended with wine and applied to the affected area will heal deadly bites. This medicine should be renewed every fourth day'.

For the mouth ~
Warm juice of verbena rolled around the mouth for a long time will ease the blisters and wounds of the mouth.

You can get the same effect by using a fresh decoction of this herb and by using this decoction foul and unpleasant breath can be sweetened - if the decoction is rolled about in the mouth so that the cheeks make a whooshing sound.

For wounds ~
This herb ground up while it is green and applied to a new wound will heal it cleanly.

For poison ~
Verbena drunk with white wine will neutralise all venoms.

For fevers ~
Take three roots of verbena and the same number of leaves and soak them in water and get the patient to drink this before he becomes ill, that is to say before he feel chilled; this drink is good for the tertian fever.

For the quartane fever take and drink 4 roots and four leaves of verbena and it will heal this fever.

A decoction of verbena made with wine and mixed with meat and drunk will make everyone merry and glad; in a similar way to Long de boef, which I have written about previously.

Place verbena in the hand of a sick person and ask him, 'how do you feel?' If he says "I think I feel better" he shall live and if he answers by saying he feels worse or says nothing, there is no hope of his life in this world.

For head aches ~
Some men have suggested that putting a corn of verbena around the aching head, whatever the cause, will quickly ease the headache.

For the bowels and the liver ~
Plinius says this herb is healing to the bowels and to the sickness of the sides and of the liver and of the thighs or breast and to the illnesses of the lungs and it also soothes coughs.

For swellings ~
Verbena ground up small with old pig fat and applied to the area will quickly ease swellings and the welkes that occur in the head through fever.

For the stone ~
Take yarrow and betony and verbena in equal quantities, grind them together and infuse them in water and drink; this is the best medicine for kidney stones that there is.

Plinius says that witches praise this herb hugely, for they say that this herb is good against all sickness and they also say that he that is anointed about with the juice of verbena should have granted him anything that they would ask. *(I interpret this to mean 'Your wishes will come true if you cover yourself in verbena juice.')*

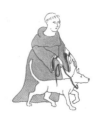

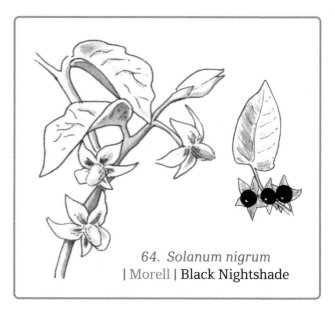

64. *Solanum nigrum*
| Morell | Black Nightshade

64.

Solanum nigrum | Morell | Black Nightshade

Morell is called in Greek *strignum* and in Latin *morella*

This is right cold

PRIMARILY

For the ear ~
It is said that the juice of this herb dropped into the ear a little at a time will ease earache.

For the leper ~
A plaster of this herb will heal leprosy and it is believed that this same plaster will heal headaches.

Inflammation of the parotid glands ~
Grind up this herb and mix it with bread and salt and make out of this a plaster and lay it onto the salivary glands ; this will ease the illness that is known as parocida. Parocida is a pustule that may develop on the salivary glands during a fever, (similar to quinsys - a suppurating infection of the tonsils).

The juice of this herb will quickly soothe 'the itch' scabies.

The juice of this herb placed onto the cervix will reduce a woman's period that is to say ease the flow of heavy periods.

For the Holy Fire/ergot poisoning ~
Grind up finely the leaves of this herb with flour and make a plaster and it will heal ergot poisoning and the evil that is known as herpes and this medicine will be significantly improved if you put into the plaster litharge of silver, ceruse (white lead) and oil of roses.

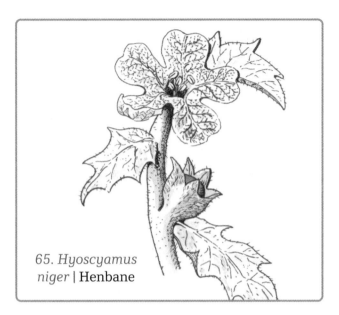

65. Hyoscyamus niger | Henbane

65.
Hyoscyamus niger | **Henbane**

This herb is said to be right cold

Of this herb there are three types:

The first has a white flower, the second brings forth a half red flower but the best produces a black flower.

The one that produces the white seed is better and nobler than the other two. But if they cannot be found, you can use the one that has the half red flower. Physicians will not work with the one that has the black flower.

PRIMARILY

For women's breasts ~
For women whose breasts ache, drink the juice of the herb that has the white flower and afterwards anoint the breasts all over with the same juice and this will ease the discomfort.

For gout ~
Grind up the leaves of this herb until they are very small together with the flowers, a plaster of this will heal all types of swellings and the hot gout.

Ears ~
This juice held in the ear will kill the worms that are present there and ease many other diseases of the ears.

Toothache ~
It is said that the vinegar in which the roots of this herb have been soaked will ease toothache even if it is very severe, the vinegar should be warm and held in the mouth for a long time.

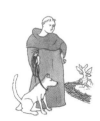

For the eyes ~
The juice wrung out of the seed of this herb when it is green, and ground up small, will heal the vicious and hot exudates that come from the eyes and burns, if the patient anoints their eyes frequently with this juice.

A scruple of this seed and also as much of poppy seed drunk together in mulsa/wine will ease haemorrhaging of the womb.

This same drink may help anyone that spits blood or for any reason bleeds from the mouth if it is drunk frequently.

Henbane seed ground up small and mixed with wine and made into a plaster will heal swollen breasts and testicles.

This herb and its seed are very valuable in plasters and medicines. But if it is eaten as a plant, it will cause the eaters to become 'wooden' this is known as mania, this will also happen if the juice is placed into an open wound.

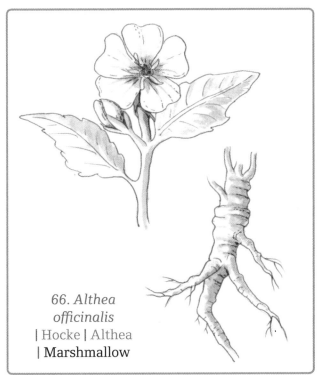

66. *Althea*
officinalis
| Hocke | Althea
| **Marshmallow**

66.
Althea
officinalis
| Hocke
| Althea
| **Marsh-**
mallow

Old men say that the
hocke is called mallow
because it makes the
womb soft.

PRIMARILY

Sextus Niger and Discorides agree that this is valuable for the
stomach and both of them say that if it is eaten as a plant it is
very healing to all parts of the body.

For poisons ~
It is very soothing for the bladder and heals the effects of all
poisonous drinks.

For wounds ~
A plaster made from mallow leaves and white willow leaves -
equal numbers of each, will heal a bleeding wound.

For bruises ~
Mallow ground up with old grease heals bruises.

Toothache ~
The root of a mallow put next to the tooth that
aches eases toothache.

Other uses ~
To avoid breast disease a woman can wear a mallow root wrapped in black wool and bound with flax to her thighs.

If goose grease is melted and mixed with the root, and then this is placed in the vagina in the form of a pessary, this will help a women deliver a dead child.

For leprosy ~
Grind mallow leaves with a little salt and this will heal the leprosy that is known as egilopa which affects the inner corner of the eye.

With mallow juice you may heal bee stings and if you mix this juice with oil and cover your body with it bees will not annoy you.

For burns ~
Warm mallow in urine and place this mixture onto the head, this will heal carbuncles and boils that form in the head and also the noxious scrofula and this plaster will ease the pain of Holy Fire and heal burns.

The decoction of mallow will soften the hardness of the uterus and help heal the causes and sicknesses of the guts and of the external opening of the ears if it is put into them.

This herb excites and causes lechery.

This is the end of the second part of Macer's book and now begins the third part which is made up of spices.

Spices

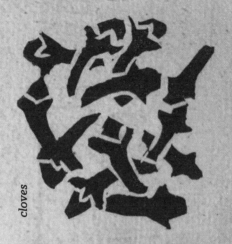

cloves

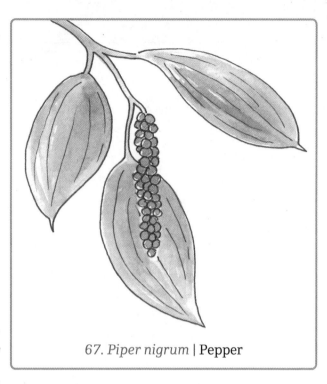

67. Piper nigrum | Pepper

67.
Piper nigrum | Pepper

Up to this point I have talked about some familiar herbs and now I'm going to look at a selection of common spices that are known to most people through their use in the kitchen but are also valuable medicines.

Pepper is hot and dry in the third degree

There are three types of pepper - white, long and black

[Here I am going to list some of the medicinal uses of black pepper]

PRIMARILY

For the stomach ~
Black pepper soaked or raw blended with honey will aid digestion, it also heals illnesses of the liver.

For bites ~
Black pepper will heal poisonous bites and ailments of the breast.

For the fever ~
This spice is particularly valuable in warming the patient suffering from periodica febris if it is taken before the trembling begins.

For gnawing in the belly ~
Grind up laurel leaves and pepper corns together and infuse in warm water. Drink this mixture to ease the gnawing in the belly.

For kernelles ~
Mix this pepper with pitch/tree resin and make the mixture into a plaster and apply this to the affected area.

For the eye ~
Mix this pepper with any other medicine that clears cataracts from the eyes and it will be more effective.

For spots ~
Mix this pepper with nitrum and make into a plaster, use this to remove any offensive spots and freckles from the face.

For cancers ~
This is one of the most useful medicines for treating cancers. Take powdered black pepper and an equivalent amount of 'man's dirt' excrement burnt to a powder, mix these together and apply this mixture to the cancer.

(My interrpretation is that you can use this pepper in almost all treatments to improve their effectiveness, it is easy to over look the value of this medicine because it is so common.)

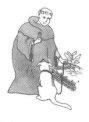

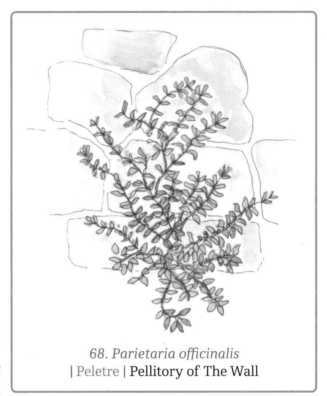

68. Parietaria officinalis
| Peletre | Pellitory of The Wall

68.
Parietaria officinalis
| Peletre
| Pellitory of The Wall

Pellitory is both hot and dry in the first degree.

PRIMARILY

For toothache ~
If a cold humour aggravates the teeth and makes them ache, chew pellitory; particularly focusing on the tooth that aches and hold it in the mouth for a long time, add to it some vinegar and roll it about the mouth, and this will help as well.

For the mouth ~
It eases swellings of the tongue that are due to excessive phlegm causing the uvula to swell up, and it also helps many other ailments of the mouth.

For epilepsy ~
If pellitory is mixed with honey it is very helpful in treating epilepsy and also the tremor associated with palsy.

It is said that if pellitory is hung around a child's neck who suffers from epilepsy this will heal him, and it will help also just by its odour alone.

For the fever ~
Anoint the body all over with the oil that pellitory has been infused in before the onset of the fever, and because of this the fever will not create as much heat as it would have done otherwise.

For the kidneys ~
This ointment will ease any aching in the kidneys.

This ointment will help to ease the palsy, if the patient is frequently rubbed vigorously with this ointment. This ointment will make the body supple and free from aches and pains.

This will bring the patient out in a hot sweat by opening up the pores.

For the lungs ~
This will also help strengthen the lungs.

The ointment will keep the body safe from the cold

For tetanus ~
Pellitory will heal the disease and contraction that is called tetanus.

Add milk to the well ground pellitory and add some oil to this mixture and apply it anywhere that needs healing and it will be very effective.

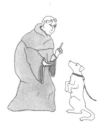

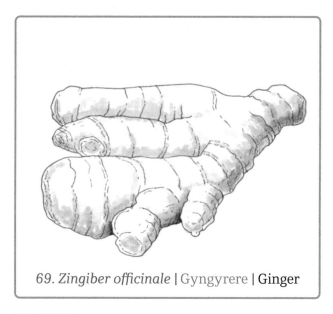

69. Zingiber officinale | Gyngyrere | Ginger

69.
Zingiber officinale | Gyngyrere | Ginger

PRIMARILY

Ginger is similar in medicine to pepper and therefore I have nothing more to add.

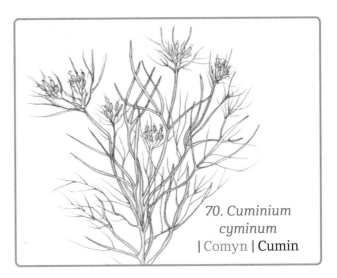

*70. Cuminium
cyminum*
| Comyn | **Cumin**

70.

*Cuminium
cyminum*
| Comyn
| **Cumin**

Cumin, as physicians
say, is both hot and dry
in the third degree.

PRIMARILY

For the stomach ~

Physicians say that cumin taken in any way will dissipate wind
that builds up in the bowel and stomach.

It increases significantly the heat of the stomach and of the
liver, and in this way improves digestion.

They say also that is destroys the lust of lechery.

For the womb ~

It will also bind the womb that is overly relaxed if the cumin is
soaked in vinegar.

Cumin drunk frequently with pusca will help ease the breathing
in orthonoyci.

For venom ~

Grind the cumin up finely and meld with bean meal and wine,
this will heal venomous bites.

For testicles ~

Cumin ground up finely and melded with honey will quickly
ease the swelling of the testicles if it is applied to the area.

Cumin drunk with pusca will reduce a woman's
period to a manageable flow.

Cumin eaten little and often will give a good
healthy colour to anyone who eats it regularly.

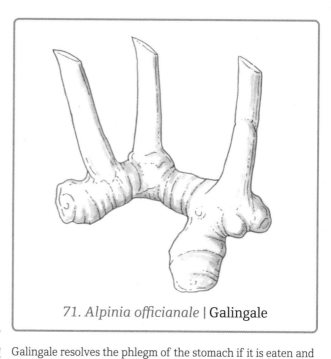

71. Alpinia officianale | Galingale

71.

Alpinia officianale | Galingale

Galingale resolves the phlegm of the stomach if it is eaten and if the patient suffers from excessive mucous it will eliminate this problem and have a strengthening effect.

PRIMARILY

For wind ~
Galingale eaten or drunk dries out wind that is closed within the bowels.

For colic ~
It helps the digestion and soothes colic.

It improves the flavour and odour of the mouth if it is eaten often.

It will also increase the lust of lechery and the heat of the kidneys if it is eaten.

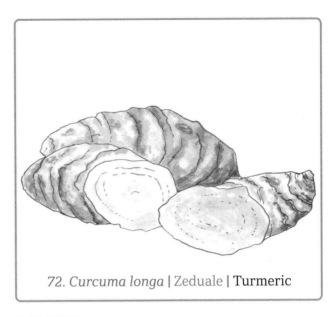

72. Curcuma longa | Zeduale | Turmeric

72. *Curcuma longa* | Zeduale | Turmeric

Turmeric is a powerful remedy against poisons found in food or drink.

PRIMARILY

For venom ~

Drink turmeric, and it will heal the bites of creeping beasties.

For the brain ~

It comforts the stomach if it is eaten often and heals diseases of the brain and puts out the noxious wind by belching and farting to enable the man to heal.

For the stomach ~

If anyone who has had a chronic digestive illness chews, after fasting, turmeric and swallows it bit by bit with his saliva, this will heal their chronic ill health.

This drink will destroy the worms of the womb and it neutralizes the stink of garlic from the mouth and also removes the great aroma of wine that accumulates in a body when a great deal of wine has been drunk.

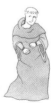

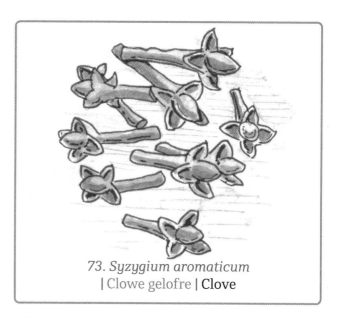

73. Syzygium aromaticum
| Clowe gelofre | Clove

73.

Syzygium aromaticum | Clowe gelofre | Clove

Clove flowers as men say are dry and hot in the second degree.

PRIMARILY

For the stomach ~
Cloves made into a decoction will comfort the stomach and the liver, and it is good for almost all the internal organs within the body.

For constipation ~
It helps wonderfully the digestion and makes the womb relaxed

A dragm weight of powder of cloves will stimulate lechery.

For the brain ~
Cloves ground small and drunk with fresh cow's milk will comfort the memory and the brain, which is the might of the mind.

74. *Cinnamomum verum*
| Canel | Cinnamon

74.
Cinnamomum verum
| Canel
| Cinnamon

Cinnamon is made up of three spices, but the best of them is the one that is most subtle and that which has the most heating effect on the tongue and also has a certain sweetness.

PRMARILY

For the stomach ~
This dries up the ill humours of the stomach and it comforts and strengthens it.

For the liver ~
Cinnamon eaten or drunk helps the liver and brings on a woman's period and makes urination easier.

For the cough ~
Cinnamon will soothe the moist cough and catarrh.

For dropsy/heart failure ~
It will ease the effect of dropsy/heart failure, which is known as tympana/distension of the abdomen due to fluid retention, and also the ache of the kidneys, and heal the bites of creeping beasties.

If cinnamon is mixed with the medicines that heal the eyes it dries up excess tear production which causes watering of the eyes.

For the face ~
Cinnamon ground very small and mixed with strong vinegar and applied as a plaster will clear the face of black spots and freckles and heal the sickness and scab known as impetigo.

For the flux ~
Grind well and small the best cinnamon and two drams of the powder drunk with cold water will staunch the bleeding of haemorrhoids, if it is drunk on an empty stomach.

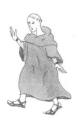

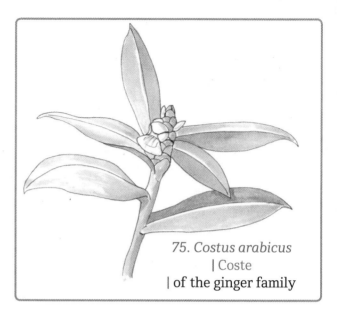

75. Costus arabicus
| Coste
| of the ginger family

75.
Costus arabicus | Coste | Of the Ginger Family

Coste has two types: one is heavy and red and comes out of India the other is light and not bitter and of a white colour; this also comes from India.

PRIMARILY

Both purge urine and eliminate anything that the body needs to release. They cure the spleen and the liver and ease the ache of the side if the patient drinks it in warm wine.

This will bring on a woman's period if the woman makes herself an infusion of this herb and drinks it, it will ease the ache of the cervix if the woman places into herself a pessary of this herb.

For the face ~
Grind this herb small with honey and this ointment will purge and clean the face of freckles and put out the worms of the belly.

This will stir lechery, if it is drunk in warm mulsa.

For the fever ~
The oil that is infused with coste when soaked in wine will prevent the cold of the fever developing if the patient is massaged with the oil before the cold come upon him.

For sciatica ~
This ointment is a sovereign medicine for sciatica and to membranes that have become numb.

For wounds ~
A powder of this herb will heal old wounds quickly.

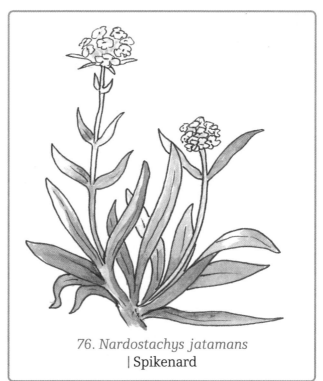

76. Nardostachys jatamans
| Spikenard

76. *Nardostachys jatamans* | Spikenard

Spikenard is hot and dry as wise men say.

PRIMARILY

For the stomach ~
A decoction of this drink comforts the liver, eases the discomforts of the stomach and purges the kidneys.

It helps the bladder and it dries up both women's periods and excess urine production.

For jaundice ~
It heals jaundice and it soothes and protects the body from the ill humours that fall from the head into the breast via the uvula.

For the intestines ~
It soothes away griping or fretting of the intestines.

For the stomach ~
Spikenard when taken as a drink will dry out the wind that is closed in the stomach, and if it is placed at the cervix it will ease the flow of blood from the uterus.

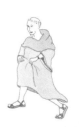

For vomiting ~

Spikenard drunk with cold water will ease the swelling of the heart and ease nausea and vomiting.

Spikenard drunk with liquor that is known as sapa will excite to lechery if it is drunk frequently.

A decoction of this will ease the hardness of the womb if the womb mouth is often sore and irritated within.

For the eyes ~

Anoint eyes frequently with this warm decoction, and it will ease the bitter itch of the eye and soothe in-growing hairs of the eye-lids, this is a very comforting and soothing treatment.

There is a type of spikenard that is known as Nardus Celtica. This grows only in the region of the people that are known as Celts, and this nard may do all that that spikenard does, though it is thought to be weaker than spikenard.

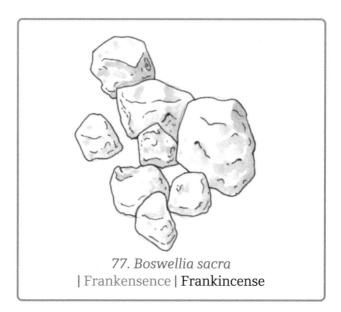

77. Boswellia sacra
| Frankensence | Frankincense

77.

Boswellia sacra

Frankensence

Frankincense

Frankincense is both hot and dry in the second degree.

PRIMARILY

For the eyes ~
Frankincense improves eyesight if it is dissolved in the white of an egg and ground up small with fresh woman's milk and applied to the eyes.

For wounds ~
Men say that frankincense ground small with vinegar and melded with pitch/wood tar and fresh milk will heal new wounds.

For burns ~
Frankincense mixed with pig fat is good for burns.

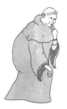

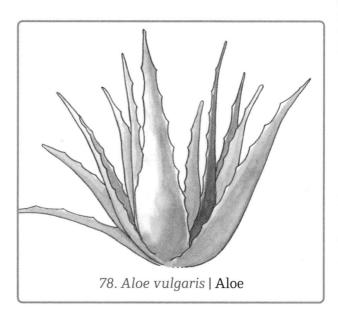

78. Aloe vulgaris | Aloe

78.
Aloe vulgaris | Aloe

There are two types of aloe, one is as red as liver, this is the colour when the leaf is broken and this is called epatice (aloe *hepatica*) and is a very valuable medicine.

The other is of a black colour when it is broken open and this has less medicinal value than the other.

PRIMARILY

For the stomach ~
Aloe cleanses the stomach of phlegm and also the head as well, it does this by purging and drying out the womb of noxious humours.

For jaundice ~
It purges the liver and helps heal jaundice.

For wounds ~
This will keep fresh wounds from rotting if a powder of this herb is sprinkled over the wound, and by drying the wound it promotes healing.

For swellings ~
This powder will particularly help reduce swellings of the womb and of the testicles.

For the lips ~
Aloe dissolved in water and laid onto the lips or nose heals the deep ulcers that sometimes develop, also it clears cloudy vision if it is applied around the eye.

For the head ~
Aloe mixed with vinegar and oil of roses will relieve headaches if the front of the head is rubbed with this mixture.

For the eyes ~
This ointment will soothe itchy eyes.

For hair ~
Aloe ground up small with wine and made into a plaster and applied to anywhere that has hairs falling out will stop this happening, where ever this maybe.

For the mouth ~
Aloe ground up small with wine and honey will help the gums, the tongue and any sores in the mouth, if it is rubbed onto the area frequently.

For the stomach ~
Aloe taken to soothe the womb will also be good for the stomach according to Vribasius, unlike all the other medicines that are used to soften the womb which irritate the stomach.

For phlegm ~
Vribasius says to take two drams of aloe with mulsa wine and it will purge both the cholera and the phlegm.

For the head ~
Anyone that is often purged using these pills will only rarely suffer from a headache.

For the eyes ~
And trust me there is nothing more profitable for the eyes than this medicine.

A laxative ~
If you want to bring on a delayed period take two parts of aloe and take one part of scammony - wild carrot and grind them well together and this mixture makes the best laxative.

Here ends the third part of the last Macer book, blessed be He of whom all good things have the beginning and end, Amen.

Now follows a few herbs of which Macer will talk about briefly so that it cannot be said that they have not been found in the course of Macer's book

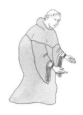

Not to be forgotten herbs

purslane

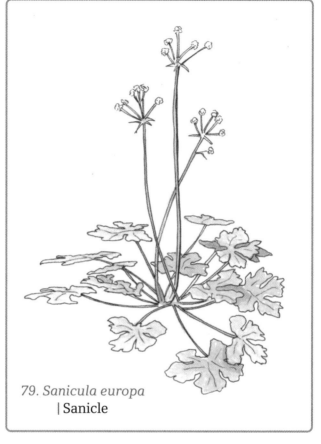

79. *Sanicula europa*
| Sanicle

79.
Sanicula europa
| Sanicle

Sanycle has her name because she heals wounds.

PRIMARILY

Wounds ~

This herb will heal both bone and flesh as the patient drinks it.

But I must be clear about how you drink this herb; because if the infection doesn't come out of the wound it will ascend into the head and into the brain and break the skin of the brain that is known as pia mater, and it will kill the patient.

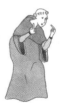

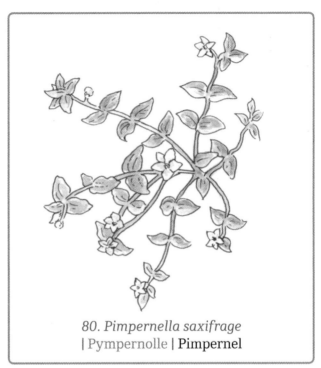

80. Pimpernella saxifrage
| Pympernolle | Pimpernel

80. *Pimpernella saxifrage* | Pymper-nolle | Pimpernel

Pimpernel grows abundantly under bushes and in the merry shadow of the woods. She has a little white flower which is black in each side.

PRIMARILY

For wounds ~
Pimpernel cleans and heals wounds.

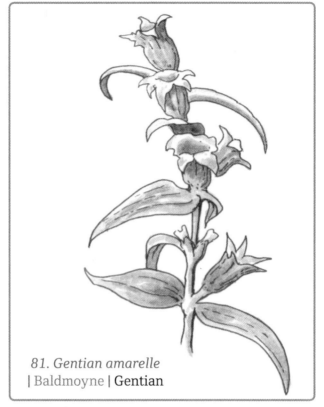

81. Gentian amarelle
| Baldmoyne | Gentian

81. *Gentian amarelle* | Baldmoyne | Gentian

PRIMARILY

Gentian helps the heart, relieves the breast and nourishes the stomach.

Gentian is found in the mire and is as effective as any bought medicine. It gives freely that which other medicines give for great price.

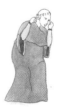

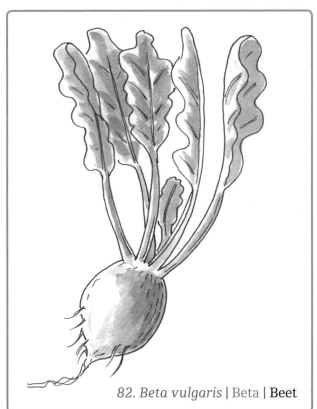

82. *Beta vulgaris* | Beta | Beet

82.
Beta vulgaris
| **Beta**
| **Beet**

PRIMARILY

Beet will quickly heal headaches and any wound in the head, and it is therefore useful as a remedy for any ailments of the head.

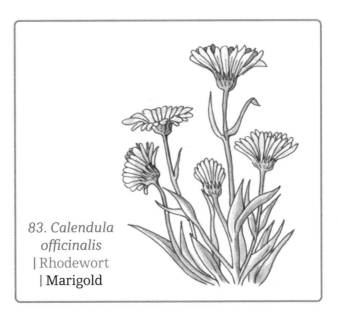

83. *Calendula officinalis*
| Rhodewort
| Marigold

83.
Calendula officinalis
| Rhodewort
| Marigold

Rodewort is known as *solsequium* in Latin and *elitropia* in Greek.

PRIMARILY

For the fever ~

This flower has great virtue, any day you see this herb the fever which is known as the acute fever will not affect you,

If you have this fever, take a leaf and a half leaf of this herb and soak it in wine and drink the wine and eat the leaves as well.

For the flux/dysentery ~

The leaves of this herb ground up finely and drunk will stop diarrhoea.

For venom ~

The juice of this herb drunk with wine will neutralise all types of venom.

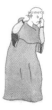

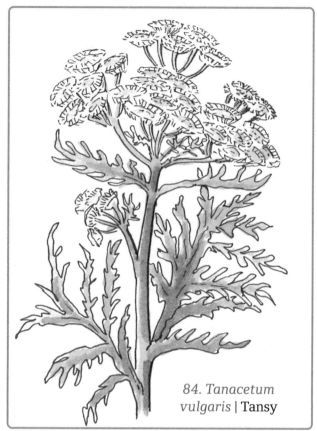

84. *Tanacetum vulgaris* | Tansy

84. *Tanacetum vulgaris* | Tansy

Thou it bite bitterly in the mouth, it is a good medicine for the breast.

PRIMARILY

For the organs in the body ~

Tansy purges not only the breast but all organs within a body. In a few words and briefly I have said and noted many virtues of this herb.

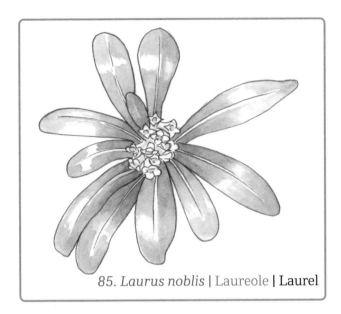

85. Laurus noblis | Laureole | Laurel

85.
Laurus noblis
| Laureole
| Laurel

PRIMARILY

Laureole is like laurel both in bark and leaves and in greenness. This herb is evergreen. It doesn't droop due to the heat of the sun, or fade in the cold. Prosius called the seed of this herb coconidion and so do many other poets and physicians. A powerful medicine can be made from this seed, which purges the bowels and heals the stomach.

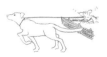

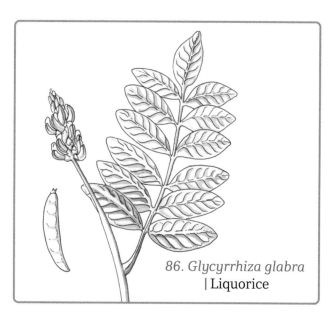

86. Glycyrrhiza glabra
| Liquorice

86.
Glycyrrhiza glabra
| **Liquorice**

Liquorice is the sweetest of all herbs.

It has a mild flavour and is extremely moist.

It is in the first degree of damp/cold or the middle of the second degree.

This is good for all illnesses and not harmful in any way, therefore she may say to mankind: 'I am your health, quickly use me'.

PRIMARILY

For the breast ~

A decoction of liquorice mixed with a stick of barley sugar when eaten will have the effect of an expectorant, soothing and moistening the sick lungs, the harsh cough, the hard and tight chest, the sore throat and the inflamed vocal cords.

There is nothing that brings up phlegm so efficiently and eases congestion of the chest as well as this medicine.

For the lungs ~

Liquorice soaked in water until it is soft and then pressed is called stick liquorice when it is dried in this way. This will soothe the lungs and ease the stiffness and diseases that affect them.

For the stomach ~

Liquorice forms a protective coating over burns and inflammations both internally and externally.

No medicine helps more effectively diseases of the lungs and chest, than does liquorice. Liquorice is very soothing, not by tormenting like Coste (see herb 75), or in irritation as does Aloe, but in gentle enjoyment.

Liquorice is the sweetest of all herbs. It is of such a mild temper that it is extremely moist. It may be in the first degree of damp/cold or the middle of the second degree. This is good for all illnesses and not harmful in any way, therefore she may say to mankind: 'I am your health, quickly use me'.

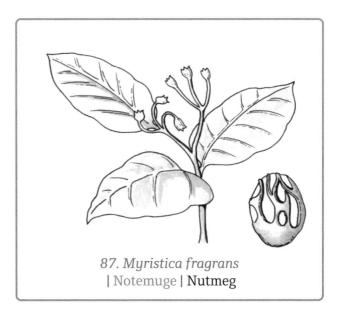

87. Myristica fragrans
| Notemuge | **Nutmeg**

87.
Myristica fragrans
| Notemuge
| **Nutmeg**

Nutmeg is both hot and dry in the second degree.

PRIMARILY

For dysentery ~
This cures bad breath, eases dysentery and prevents heavy periods: it strengthens both the liver and the stomach.

For the liver ~
Galen said that the nutmeg makes the skin fair, it cures the spleen and reduces the swellings of the liver.

This will soothe and ease gout, and, it is said, it will heal wounds quickly.

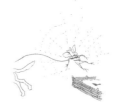

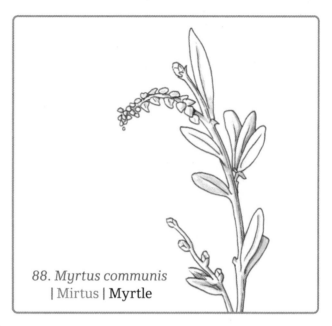

88. Myrtus communis
| Mirtus | Myrtle

88.
Myrtus communis | Mirtus | Myrtle

Myrtle is abundant in the far north. It grows happily in the cold.

Myrtle is hot in flavour.

PRIMARILY

For the bloody dysentery ~

Make a decoction of myrtle and mix it with the juice of plantain in equal parts and heat them together. This will heal the bloody dysentery and the sickness that is a kind of chronic flux of the intestines. If you feel that you need something stronger consider using oak apples.

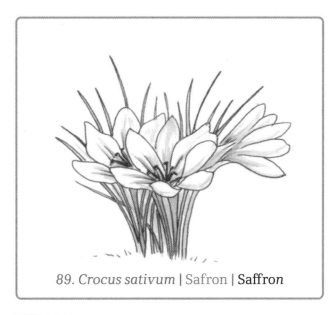

89. *Crocus sativum* | Safron | **Saffron**

89.
Crocus sativum
| Safron
| **Saffron**

Saffron is very healing to many illnesses.

PRIMARILY

For the eyes ~
Saffron flowers mixed with a mother's milk and kept for a while will heal sore eyes if it is applied to the eyes, it also neutralises venom.

For sciatica ~
Mix together saffron, frankincense and cokill *(Interestingly Lolium temulentum is often affected by the ergot fungus, another name for this plant is poison grass)*. Warm them together in mulsa wine and place onto the place that is affected and this will heal sciatica.

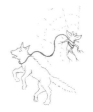

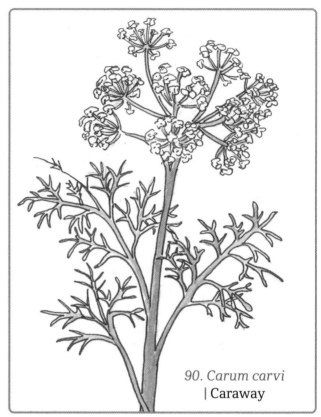

90. *Carum carvi*
| Caraway

90.
Carum carvi
| Caraway

Caraway is hot and sharp in flavour.

Caraway and chervil are similar in colour, shape and medicinal uses.

The leaves are cerule in colour as are the leaves of chervil. Ceruleus is yellow similar to wax or green and black mixed together as when yellow is seen with black in the way caraway leaves look, chervil leaves have a similar appearance.

PRIMARILY

This herb encourages lechery and also increases urination.

It also brings on a woman's period and has a pleasant flavour and taste.

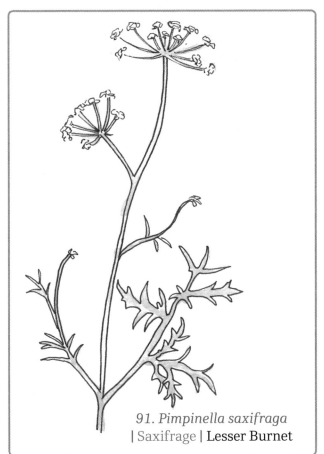

91. Pimpinella saxifraga
| Saxifrage | **Lesser Burnet**

91. *Pimpinella saxifraga* | Saxifrage | **Lesser Burnet**

Saxifrage has a reputation for breaking and dissolving kidney stones. Some call it *petroselinum*.

PRIMARILY

For the stone ~

Grind together saxifrage and cherry stones and give this as a drink in hot water to dissolve kidney stones. People say that there is no better medicine for dissolving kidney stones than this, but this will only be effective if the stone is small and has only recently developed. If the stone has been there for a long time then it must be dissolved with a stronger medicine,

For the fever ~

Physicians have said that saxifrage is helpful to anyone who has a fever.

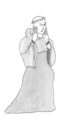

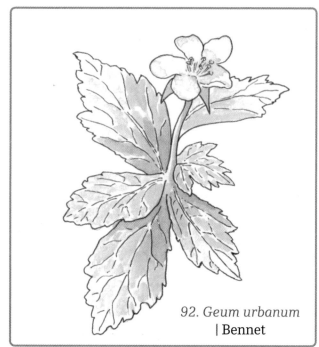

92. *Geum urbanum*
| Bennet

92.
Geum urbanum
| Bennet

Bennet is called hare's ear.

PRIMARILY

For wounds ~
This will cleanse a wound and afterwards fill it with good flesh of a healthy pink colour and it is good for gout.

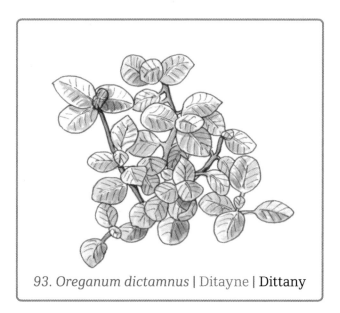

93. Oreganum dictamnus | Ditayne | Dittany

93.
Oreganum dictamnus | Ditayne | Dittany

Dittany is used abundantly in soup.

PRIMARILY

Virgil wrote that Aeneas was wounded with an arrow. When it could not be removed he put dittany into the wound and this poultice brought out the arrow. In this way Virgil has passed on the information that dittany will bring out iron from a wound that cannot be pulled out with tools.

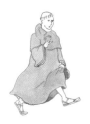

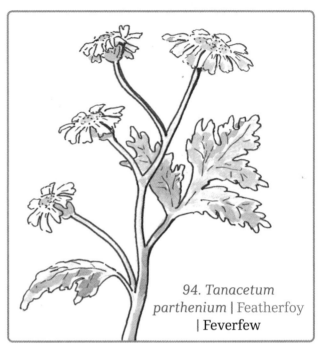

94. *Tanacetum parthenium* | Featherfoy | Feverfew

94.
Tanacetum parthenium | Featherfoy | Feverfew

PRIMARILY

Featherfoy is a known as a febrifuge, she will reduce and cool bitter fevers and therefore the name reflects this.

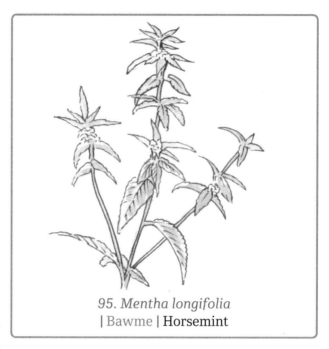

95. *Mentha longifolia*
| Bawme | Horsemint

95.
Mentha longifolia
| Bawme
| Horsemint

Horsemint is very beautiful with a pleasant flavour and a sweet fragrance. This is known sometimes as *ciralis*, sometimes *simbria*.

PRIMARILY

For fever ~
Give the patient two scripulus of this to drink in hot water.

For the bladder ~
If you have a disease in the bladder, or if you have that evil that is caused by an enlarged prostate, so that a man often has difficulty in urinating, then drink the juice of this with wine and you will be healed.

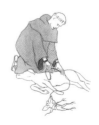

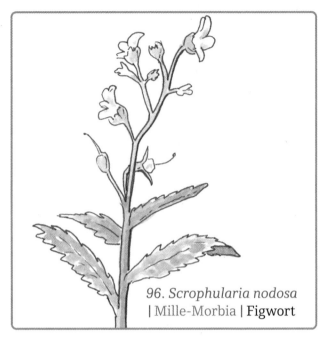

96. *Scrophularia nodosa* | Mille-Morbia | Figwort

96.

Scrophularia nodosa | Mille-Morbia | Figwort

Mille-mawbia is medicinal to a thousand sicknesses and also is known by many other names.

PRIMARILY

For wounds ~

This is as good for healing wounds as comfrey and in some cases is even more effective than comfrey.

For the eye ~

In a similar way to rue this herb clears and sharpens the eye-sight.

For gout ~

This is very effective in healing the extremely fierce and violent gout.

For venom ~

Salix alba - white willow eases pain no better than this herb. What else can I tell you about this herb? It has virtues without number.

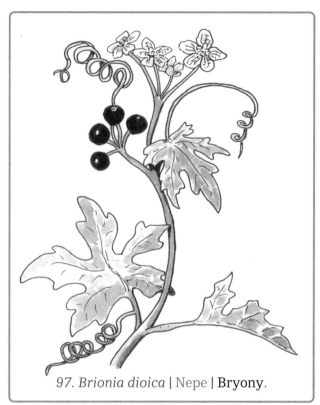

97. Brionia dioica | Nepe | Bryony.

97.
Brionia dioica | Nepe | Bryony

Nepe is known in Latin Raphanus

PRIMARILY

For cancer ~

This herb can help in treating cancer but there is a process that has to be followed first:

First bind a frog to the cancer overnight; this will effectively consume and dry up the cancer in a way that you will wonder at, by the following day the skin will be amazingly dry. Then take away the frog and apply to the area a mixture of bryony root, cow urine and rye flour, this will take away all the strength and might of the cancer leaving only an open wound. Then treat the wound as you would heal any other wound.

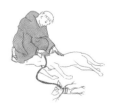

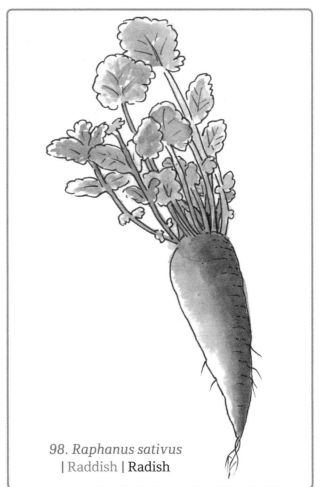

98.
Raphanus sativus
| Raddish
| **Radish**

Radish has the same or similar virtues to bryony but it is a little weaker.

98. *Raphanus sativus*
| Raddish | **Radish**

PRIMARILY

This is good to increase urination.

For the breast ~
This is a tonic to the breast and to the organs of the body.

Whoever eats this herb root in the time that Mars reigns, it will lengthen his life.

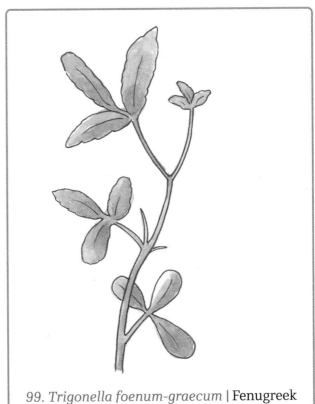

99. *Trigonella foenum-graecum* | Fenugreek

99.
Trigonella foenum-graecum | Fenugreek

PRIMARILY

Fenugreek will soften swellings and abscesses and ease the tightening of tissues or ligaments; it will do this if used by itself, but it will do it more effectively if it is used with wild mallow.

For encasema/ a small red growth forming at the inner corner of the eye.

A plaster of fenugreek and cabbage ground up finely with vinegar will make arthritic conditions more comfortable it will also be beneficial for gout; this plaster may make the sufferers of arthritis and gout lithe and supple.

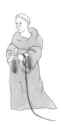

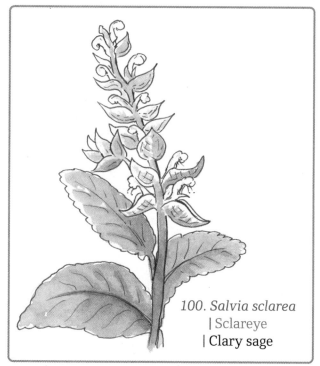

100. *Salvia sclarea*
| Sclareye
| Clary sage

100.
Salvia sclarea
| Sclareye
| Clary Sage

Clary sage is good for the hot gout.

PRIMARILY

For the voice ~

Clary sage clarifies the voice that has been hoarse and has a very healing effect on the lungs and the liver and the bowel; and there are many other virtues to this herb which wise physicians use it for.

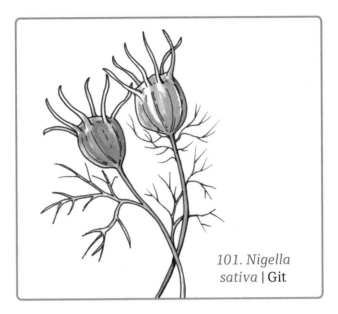

*101. Nigella
sativa* | Git

101.
*Nigella
sativa*
| **Git**

PRIMARILY

Git has four corners or pikes or horns growing upwards, if you add these four corners or 'horns' to bread it will improve the flavour immeasurably. Git is also good and precious for many other reasons and purposes.

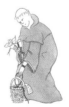

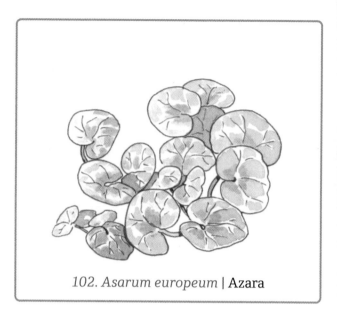

102. Asarum europeum | Azara

102.

Asarum europeum | **Azara**

Azara may be called a tree in comparison to other small herbs, and a herb in comparison to a tree.

PRIMARILY

For the body ~
This herb will ease aches and pains that occur in the body.

Grind up the roots of this herb until they are very small, mix with wine and drink, this will soon cause great vomiting and cure the illness. But only use this medicine when you can see that all other medicines have failed to effect a cure, because this is a great and a strong medicine. *(In my opinion also a dangerous medicine).*

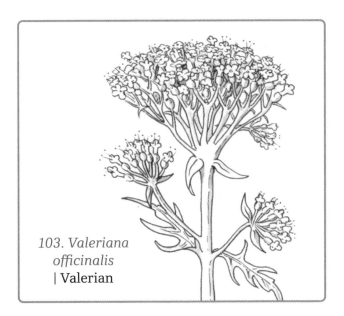

*103. Valeriana
officinalis*
| Valerian

103.
*Valeriana
officinalis*
| **Valerian**

PRIMARILY

Valerian has great value, she has a large flowering top and small seeds. A piece of valerian herb or seeds ground up finely is good and healing for many illnesses.

For the fever ~
This soaked in wine and drunk will heal you of the fever

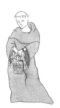

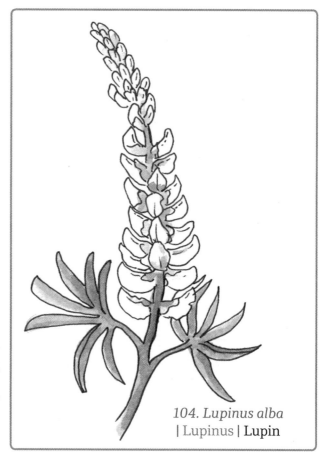

104. *Lupinus alba*
| Lupinus | Lupin

104.
Lupinus alba
| Lupinus
| Lupin

PRIMARILY

Lupin is a herb that grows with the beans in the field. It has large sharp prickles; whoever eats this in potage will not be drunk for long.

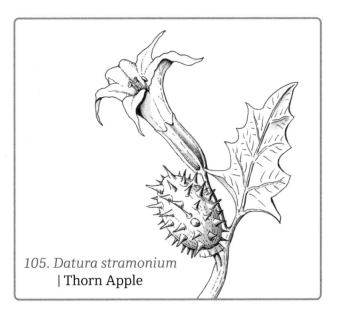

105. Datura stramonium
| Thorn Apple

105.
Datura stramonium
| Thorn Apple

PRIMARILY

For dysentery ~
This cures bad breath, eases dysentery and prevents heavy periods: it strengthens both the liver and the stomach.

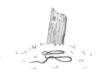

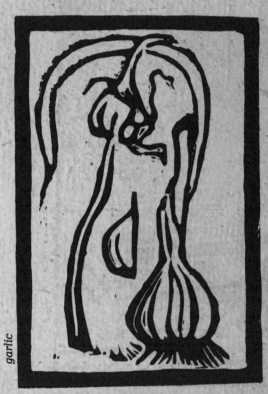

garlic

*Atropa
mandragora*
| Mandragora
Satan's Apple
| Mandrake

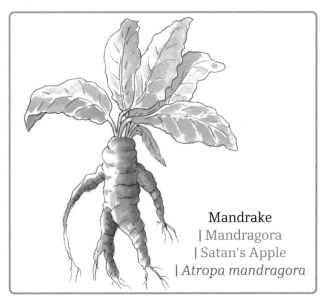

Mandrake
| Mandragora
| Satan's Apple
| *Atropa mandragora*

Family - solanacea

Mandrake has been linked to many strange ideas and superstitions over the centuries.

It will grow successfully in the European climate as long as it is protected from frost, Turner (author of the Niewe Herball) is recorded as growing it in 1562.

It has a large root that often divides into 3 or four branches - these can take on the appearance of the limbs and trunk of a man or woman. The leaves may grow up to a foot in length and have a musty feotid aroma, the flowers are bell shaped, white with a pinkish tinge and the fruit is small and round with a yellow colour when ripe with a strange apple like scent.

Medicinal Uses

The leaves are cooling and historically when boiled in milk were used as a poultice for chronic ulcers.

The fresh root has a powerful purgative and emetic effect. It was considered to have pain killing properties and a soothing, calming effect on the patient. In large doses it was said to cause delirium and madness. Mandrake root was used to allow a patient in severe pain to sleep, it was also considered effective in treating melancholy, convulsions, rheumatic pains and tumours.

The part that was used predominately was the bark of the root - either by expressing the juice or infusing the bark in water. The root grated into a pulp and mixed with brandy - was considered most effective in treating the chronic pain of rheumatism.

Mandrake was used in Pliny's time and although some of the contents of Macer are considered to derive from the writings of Pliny, mandrake is not mentioned in Macer. Pliny reports that mandrake was used as a general anaesthetic before an operation was carried out - a piece of the root was given to the patient to chew causing drowsiness and the ability to withstand pain.

Legends

In Anglo Saxon herbals mandrake was considered to have mystical powers and the ability to drive out demons from people who were considered to be posessed.

Bartholomew is one source of the old mandrake legend: 'the rind melded with wine and given to them as a drink that shall be cut in their body will not feel the pain of the saw.'

Uprooting the mandrake:

When uprooting a mandrake plant the digger must beware of contrary winds and also he must keep on digging until sunset.

Owing to the roots of mandrake resembling the human form they were often drawn in the old herbals as male - with a long beard or female - with a bushy head of hair.

The plant was said to be found growing under gallows where murderers had been hanged.

'It was considered to be death to dig up the root which was said to utter a shriek or terrible groans on being dug up, which none may hear and live. It was held, therefore, that he who would take up a plant of mandrake should tie a dog to it for that purpose, who drawing it out would certainly perish, as the man would have done, had he attempted to dig it up in the ordinary manner'.

In Henry VIII's time images of people were carved from Bryony roots and passed off as being from mandrake roots, they were called puppettes or mammettes and were supposed to have magical powers.

Source - A Modern Herbal Mrs M. Grieve

For a visual experience o uprooting the mandrake please flick through the pages of this book and watch carefully the bottom right hand corne

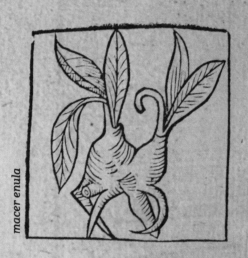

macer enula

Soutra hospital research project excavations

Life saving remedies and treatments from Soutra's past

The trenches and cellars that make up the drains of Soutra

SHARP (Soutra Hospital Archaeological Research Project) Brian Moffat has produced six volumes since 1988 based on what lies in the cellars, drains and trenches found at Soutra. The following pages show a layout of the hospital where the excavations took place with details of what was found in each area. There are cross references to the key Macer Floribus herb texts.

To learn more you can write to Brian Moffat at: Corstorphine High St Edinburgh, EH12 7SY

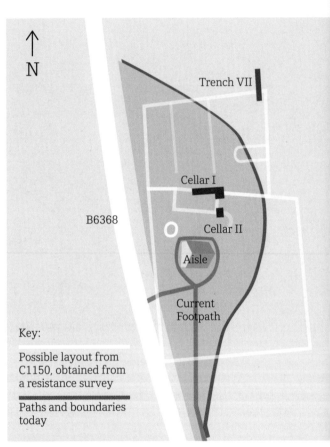

Key:

Possible layout from C1150, obtained from a resistance survey

Paths and boundaries today

Excavations

Excavated drains at Soutra include:
Trench VII
Cellar I
Cellar II

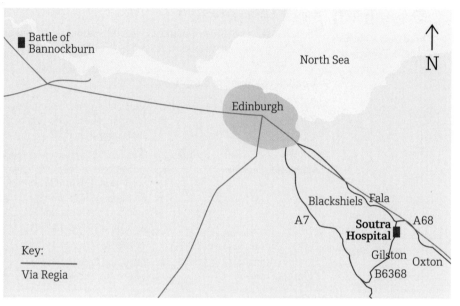

The complex at Soutra was built close to the Via Regia, the main route from the North to the Abbeys on the Scottish borders. The hospital was known as the House of the Holy Trinity, and was run by the Augustinian Order and is believed to have been the largest hospital in medieval Scotland.
Source: James Hunter 1892.

The Battle of Bannockburn took place a few miles from the site of Soutra and it is very posisble that casualties from the battlefield would have been brought to Soutra Hospital.

The bulk of the information from the excavations at Soutra comes from the drains that were linked to the infirmary.

above: area map
previous page: site map

Trench VII

Three sub-samples from Trench VII

Sample 1 from Trench VII

These consist of masses of material with indications of degraded blood. No pollen is present in this sample which included some birch charcoal.

A pollen count from 6.5g clay:

Myrtle species / *Myrtus communis*	64 grains	This has a powerful binding effect on the bowels due to its high tannin content
Mugwort / *Artemisia vulgaris*	16 grains	Although Macer considered it to be predominately used as a woman's herb in this context its purpose was probably to 'comfort the stomach' and act as a tonic to the digestive system
Plantain / ribwort / *Plantago major*	3 grains	Soothing and healing internally and externally
Composites with 'latex'	3 grains (latex from opium?)	Pain relief

Lead content of the clay matrix was 10 times higher in some areas than others, possible site of lead pipes.

SHARP Practice Volume 2 1988

This mixture was probably made up to treat someone suffering from the 'bloody flux' a purging, painful diarrhoea.

Sample 2 from Trench VII

Residues found on six shards:

The shards are coarse, thick and crudely glazed in a yellow/greenish colour probably southern Scottish C14. They were incorporated in the primary fill/open drain.

Opium poppy / *Papaver somniferum*	13 grains	Pain relief
Corn poppy / *Papaver rhoeas*	1 grain	Possibly contamination although this poppy was used for treating mild pain, coughs and insomnia.
Chickweed family / *Stellaria media*	2 grains	Although not mentioned in Macer this herb is found throughout Britain and is used particularly for its soothing effect on the digestive tract and externally for itchy skin conditions.
Plantain/Ribwort / *Plantago major*		Soothing and healing
Charred cereal grains	An over cooked meal? Porridge	A method of administering the herbs?

This mixture would have been very gentle and soothing, the fact that it was found on shards of pottery may indicate that it had been stored in a container for external use.

By 1989,
99 pollen analyses
had been completed
on excavated material
from Soutra

Sample 3 from Trench VII

8 pollen analyses have proved to be related to the general environment of Trench VII, an open drain.

28 are evidently swamped by certain cultivated plants:

Hemp / a variety of *Cannabis sativa*	9 pollen spores	Calming and relaxing / anthelmintic / worms / parasites
Flax / *Linum usitissimum*	3 pollen spores	Bulk laxative also used as a poultice externally
Hemp with flax	6 pollen spores	A blend of the actions above
Opium poppy / *Papaver somniferum*	4 pollen spores	Calming also relieves pain
Cereal coupled with micro remains of *Avena sativa*	6 bristle oats	Possibly the basis of a meal or a drink - the oats would have had a calming and relaxing effect on the nervous system and are very nutritious.

A further 9 have a substantial presence of cultivated plants often assorted.

A further 6 were taken from hearth waste to ascertain the woody species.

31 are reasonably certain to be residues of the former contents of pottery vessels.

SHARP Practice
Volume 3 1989

The remaining 17 are yet to be identified.

Other plant material discovered there:

Tormentil / *Potentilla erecter*	A herb often administered in porridge as a means of worming people in the spring - spring cleaning
Hemp / a variety of *Cannabis sativa*	Relaxing sedative and anthelmintic / wormer
Cultivated flax / *Linum usitatissimum*	The seed can be used as a bulk laxative, a poultice or as an anthelmintic.
Opium poppy / *Papaver somniferum*	Sedative, pain relief

A relaxing blend which would also eliminate parasites.

Hemp was used to treat plague, poison, tumours and abscesses, gout, crossbow wounds, dislocated joints, 'fester' and 'cancre'.

Scotia Illustrata 1684 by Sir Robert Sibbald (joint founder of the Royal College of Physicians of Edinburgh and the Physic Garden), gives the uses of these herbs:

Hemp / a variety of *Cannabis sativa* (seed and juice)	Anthelmintic / worms / parasites
Cannabis sativa	Diarrhoea and flux
Flax / *Linum usitatissimum*	Tumours, bulk laxative - treatment for constipation
Opium poppy / *Papaver somniferum*	Narcotic, relaxing, pain relief

Hemp and flax were also grown and used to make cloth.

Cellar I

Medical waste found at Soutra near the south wall

SHARP Practice
Volumn 4 1992

Appendices

The Soutra ointment jar recovered from Cellar I

This jar held a grease based ointment containing traces of:

Opium poppy / *Papaver somniferum* - narcotic

A variety of Hemp / *Cannabis sativa* - anthelmintic / worms

Myrrh / *Commophora molmol* - antiseptic / antibacterial

Rose / *Rosa damascena* - soothing and cooling

Cedar / *Cedrus libanus* - anti bacterial / anti viral

It was possibly a treatment for alleviating pain due to the presence of the opium and hemp and would also have had a soothing antiseptic effect due to the myrrh, rose and cedar.

Possibly a treatment for alleviating the symptoms of Holy Fire.

First medical waste discovery, identified from Cellar I Cache of 574 seeds:

372 seeds - Black henbane / *Hyoscymus niger*

94 seeds - Hemlock / *Conium maculatum*

108 seeds - Opium poppy / *Papaver somniferum*

SHARP Practice
Volume 5 1995

The classic mixture of henbane, opium and hemlock is, as we know, the basis for a medieval general anaesthetic and this mixture has been found a number of times during this excavation which indicates that it was used on a regular basis. Also the remnant of a heel bone that was found in this part of the excavation is proof that surgery of some kind was being performed on this site.

Second medical waste discovery, identified from Cellar I

11 rye seeds - Ergot / *Claviceps purpurea* on Secale cereale
- mixed with a mixture of Juniper berries / *Juniperus communis*
and twigs - was this possibly an aid to childbirth?

Watercress / *Nasturtium officinale* mixed with liver fluke ova
plus tooth - treatment for loose teeth, scurvy?
(liver fluke - unintentional addition)

15 whip worm ova & 4 maw worm ova - were these the results of
one of the anthelmintic treatments mentioned?

20cm long bone from an infant

Appendices

Ergot / *Claviceps purpurea* - A powerful antihaemorrhagic for
use particularly during childbirth to stem haemorrhaging used
today in the form ergotamine.

Juniper / *Juniperus communis* - A powerful herb with anti
bacterial properties often used to treat urinary tract infections.
It also has a stimulating effect on the uterus which promotes child
birth, the delivery of the afterbirth or the delivery of a preterm
foetus.

These herbs found together indicate that they were probably
used as an aid to child birth or to ensure the delivery of the
afterbirth/placenta.

Watercress / *Nasturtium officinale* - A green vegetable high in
vitamins and minerals particularly vitamin C.

Liver fluke ova / *Fasciola hepatica* - Liver fluke is a hazard of
eating watercress. Part of its life cycle involves spending time
either on grass or other green plants before being eaten, usually by
sheep. Its inclusion with the watercress is certainly accidental, it
would have caused liver damage in its new host.

Appendices *continued*

Second medical waste
discovery, identified
from Cellar I

Tooth - This was found wrapped in the watercress, loose teeth can be an early sign of scurvy (a lack of vitamin C, causing spongy gums, loosening of the teeth and bleeding into the tissues causing the appearance of bruises). Treating this condition with a herb that contains good levels of vitamin C would have begun to reverse the condition within a few days; although the connection between scurvy and fresh fruit and vegetables would not be formally recognised until the navy began to issue citrus fruit to sailors in 1800 AD. The consumption of fresh fruit and vegetables was not a priority during medieval times and would not be until C18. There was limited availability of fresh fruit and vegetables especially during the hungry gap between January and June, until preserving, bottling, salting, freezing and importing fresh food became possible.

Whip and maw worm ova - parasitic worms would have been a normal feature in the average person's gut flora during the medieval period. When Richard lll's remains were discovered the ova of a round worm was found alongside his skeleton. In Macer there are many references to anthelmintics - herbs that 'expel worms from the belly'.

20cm long bone from an infant - The reason for the presence of this bone in the drains at Soutra can only be subject to speculation. Possibly due to amputation or the death of an infant with this being the only remnant. It does indicate that the patients in the infirmary at Soutra were not exclusively male, we have seen that women may have been among the patients and this discovery indicates that children were patients as well.

Excavation sample from Cellar I

1. 16 Secale cereale / Ergot spurs mixed with 100-120 Juniper berries / *Juniperus communis*, plus twigs

2. 238 seeds of Watercress / *Rorippa nasturtium-aquaticum* also 34 seeds from 14 species of assorted aquatic plant species

3. 386 Sweet cicely / *Myrrhis odorata* seeds close to 614 seeds of Bistort / *Persicaria bistorta*

4. 573 seeds of Coltsfoot / *Tussilago farfara*, 36 seeds of Liquorice / *Glycyrrhiza glabra* with 3 root fragments of liquorice and 3 filaments of Saffron / *Crocus sativus* pressed into one of the pieces of liquorice root

5. 146 seeds of Valerian / *Valeriana officianalis* mixed with 48 seeds of Nettle / *Urtica doica* and St. Johns Wort / *Hypericum perforatum*

6. Fragment of Nutmeg / *Myristica fragrans* and 11 Mistletoe seeds / *Viscum album*

7. Fragment of human heel bone which lies over a mass of wood tar.

Appendices

1. Again we see the mixture of ergot and juniper.

2. Watercress – see page XXXIX.

3. Dr Moffat had a nutritional profile done on both these herbs at The Scottish Agricultural College, Auchincruive. This showed a good range of minerals and some vitamins present in both plants, the most remarkable findings were unexpectedly high levels of selenium in sweet cicely 5.0 ug/100g as opposed to 1.5ug/100g in bistort. Both plants also had useful levels of iron, manganese, potassium, boron, zinc and calcium.

4. Coltsfoot / *Tussilago farfara* **and Liquorice /** *Glycyrrhiza glabra* **and Saffron /** *Crocus sativus* – these herbs throughout history have been used to treat coughs and chest infections as well as other conditions although saffron has fallen out of current medicinal use.

5. Valerian/ *Valeriana officianalis*, **Nettles/***Urtica doica* **and St. John's Wort/***Hypericum perforatum*
Valerian has a calming effect without causing drowsiness and St. John's Wort is uplifting and has been proved to be useful in treating mild to moderate depression. Nettles are currently used as a tonic, in recent history the Physio Medicalists called it a 'blood cleanser. Excellent for treating gout, itchy skin conditions and high blood pressure although nettles also contain serotonin which may have been the reason for including them in this mixture.

6. Fragment of nutmeg/*Myristica fragrans* **and mistletoe/***Viscum album* **seeds**
Both of these herbs have a relaxing effect. Nutmeg has a soothing effect on the digestive system. These are relatively gentle herbs and might have been used to soothe digestive and emotional upsets. Although mistletoe is used today in the form of small twigs and leaves, the seeds are considered toxic.

7. Fragment of human heel bone – there are unusual facies and ridges on this calcaneum which may indicate a club foot. The wood tar might have been applied to stop the bleeding and/or to cover the exposed area until granulation/healing had become established.

Cellar II

Beneath cellar II

Juniper / *Juniperus communis*	3cm diameter charred berries	Antiseptic smoke, perhaps used to purify the air in the infirmary
Sweet cicely / *Myrrhis odorata*	386 seeds	High in selenium, boosts the immune system and fertility
Valerian / *Valeriana officinalis* Nettles / *Urtica doica*	146 seeds	Calming tonic
Bistort / *Bistorta officinalis*	614 seeds	Mixed with porridge as a wormer/anthelmintic. Also anti-haemorrhagic.

Appendices

Beneath cellar II

Juniper/*Juniperus communis* - 3cm diameter piece of charred wood. Producing fragrant, possibly anti bacterial, smoke which would overlay other, less pleasant odours in the infirmary.

Sweet cicely/*Myrrhis odorata* seeds - These are warming to the digestive system which encourages flatulence to dissipate. High in selenium they also boost the immune system and fertility.

Valerian/ *Valeriana officianalis* - According to Macer this herb was used to treat fevers. A very common herb around Soutra it is also extremely effective at reducing anxiety, an anti-depressant which does not cause tiredness. This is a herb which could have been used regularly in a war zone such as the border country.

Nettles/*Urtica dioca* - Nettles are one of nature's great tonics they contain high levels of vitamin C, chlorophyll, histamine, iron, calcium and silica as well as serotonin. Good serotonin levels are important for feeling 'happy'; low levels are associated with depression. Macer has a number of uses for nettles particularly for lung health.

This mixture of valerian and nettles suggests that it was used as a calming, uplifting tonic.

Bistort/*Bistorta officianalis* (Easter Ledges) - The root is extremely astringent and could have been used to treat diarrhoea. The leaves (and possibly seeds) are the main ingredient in Easter Ledge pudding - a boil in the bag barley pudding including a selection of spring greens including dandelion leaves, black currant leaves, goose grass and nettles. This is a meal that would often be prepared around Easter time to celebrate spring and the new availability of fresh green vegetables - a much needed opportunity to consume some vitamin C as well as other trace elements.

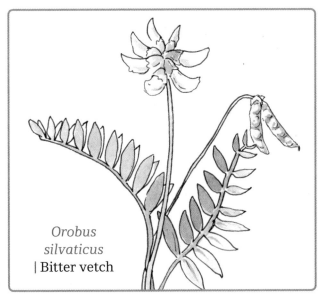

Orobus
silvaticus
| Bitter vetch

Other plant material
found in the drains:

Orobus
silvaticus
| **Bitter Vetch**
| Carmele
| Carameile
| Heath pea
| Lathyrus
macrorhizus

SHARP Practice
volume 6 1998
Brian Moffat

Bitter Vetch / *Orobus silvaticus*
Carmele, Carameile, the heath pea - Lathyrus macro rhizus.

Tourists travelling through Scotland in the C17 and C18 mention the use of bitter vetch tubers or heath pea rhizomes.

James Robertson (possibly Scotland's first ethnobotanist) in 1768 wrote in his journal 'they (the peasants/crofters) eat the roots of the Orobus tuberosus or cart mel; they eat this when they are thirsty or famished.'

Lightfoot 1792:
"I have often seen it dried and kept for journeys through hills where no provisions were to be had."

Sir Robert Stibbald, Physician, botanist and author of 'Provision For The Poor In Times Of Dearth And Scarcity'.

"Our highlanders (which are of the race of the Ancient Britons) to preserve them from hunger and thirst make much use of the knobs upon the roots of the karemyle which is the orobus silvaticus, the round knobs have the taste of liquorice; they keep it in their mouth the bigness of a bean or pease; they infuse it too in the water they drink, and they make a drink of the decoction of the knobs of it; in the strength of this they can travel and toil."

Bitter vetch continued   **Hector Boece**:

"In extreme hunger they used it when they did want for all other provisions and by sucking it they appeased their appetite and sustained their life, and this might be of great use to the poor now and their young ones in their extremity."

It appears that somehow the root of the bitter vetch was able to allay thirst and hunger thereby allowing poor crofters to survive the hungry gap before the introduction of the potato, which allowed them to grow enough food to store throughout the winter.

When this information filtered through to London it created great excitement from the navy who tried to carry out an experiment to see if it could cut down on rations for seamen by feeding them the root of the heath pea - they mutinied.

Nell Gwynn was also fascinated by the possibilities of this simple root and used it to lose weight.

Despite these attempts to harness the potential of this plant the heath pea fell out of favour with entrepreneurs but continued to be used by crofters in the highlands of Scotland.

A history of medieval anaesthesia:

The school in Salerno was the first school in Europe which taught medicine to outsiders or lay people who were not members of the religious foundation. Previously this medical knowledge was passed on from experienced monks to novices.

The school was established in the 9th century in a Benedictine community and reached its apogee in the 12th century.

A recipe for a general anaesthetic mixture is attributed to 12th century writings from Salerno - this recipe includes opium (Papava somniferum), henbane (Hyocymus niger), poppy seeds (Papava somniferum), ivy (Hedera helix), mulberries (morus niger), lettuce (lactuca virosa) and hemlock (Conium maculatum (Brandt 1997).

Roger Frugardi in Practica Chirugiae, (1471) and Nicolas Prepositus (Dean of the Salerno school) in Antidotary 1471 describe a soporific sponge formula. The mixture used is likely to have been developed by Arab physicians as many medical works were translated at the Benedictine Abbey of Monte Cassino.

Although Christian physicians used alcohol as a sedative, clearly Islamic physicians would not have had this option and needed to develop an alternative.

Constantinus Africanus (1015 -1087) worked at the school at Salerno translating Arab sources and also texts from Hypocrates and Galen. His writings were translated into Latin, probably by Abbot Bertharius, one of the translations mentions a soporific sponge - this is one of the oldest medicinal recipes known to date.

For a soporific sponge:

"Take of Opium and the juice of morus (mulberry), Hyocymus niger (henbane), the juice of Conium maculatum (hemlock), the juice of leaves of mandragora (mandrake), juice of Hedera helix (climbing ivy), of Lactuca virosa (lettuce seed), and of the seed of lapathum (dock), which has round hard berries and of Cicuta maculata (water hemlock) one ounce of each.

Mix all these together in a brazen vessel and then put into it a new sponge. Boil all together out in the sun during the dog days, until all is consumed and cooked down into the sponge. As often as there is need, you may put this sponge into hot water for an hour and apply it to the nostrils until the subject for the operation falls asleep. Then the surgery may be performed and when it is completed in order to wake him up soak another sponge in vinegar and pass it frequently under his nostrils. For the same purpose place the juice of fennel root in his nostrils soon he will awaken." (Reworked translation) This was taken from 'Infusino', a review of medieval recipies for the soporific sponge. O'Neill & Calmes 1989.

Twelve recipes have been recorded mentioning the soporific sponge in medieval writings and although the mixtures vary slightly the main ingredients remain the same. (Brunn 1928: Kuhlen 1983).

Alternative methods of medieval anaesthesia:

"A drynke that men callen dwale to make a man slepe whyle men kerven hem." 'A drink called dwale: a surgical anaesthetic used in late medieval England' (Voigts L.E. & Hudson R.P. 1992).

The classic ingredients of dwale include: pig bile - bore for a man, sow for a woman, hemlock, bryony or mandrake - depending on availability, lettuce, opium and henbane. This mixture was drunk by the patient until they fell asleep - this would allow the appropriate dose to be taken by the patient. The antidote was vinegar which would be used to wash the face of the patient - they would revive 'instantly', this part of the process is very similar to reviving the patient after using the soporific sponge.

Paracelsus 1493-1541, considered to be the father of chemical medicine, developed his own recipe for a general anaesthetic using similar ingredients to these medieval sources: Theban opium, cinnamon, musk/ambergris, poppy seeds, mandrake root, mastic resin and henbane juice.

Ultimately these mixtures were replaced by the use of laudanum and other opium derivatives, safer for the patient but highly addictive.

The main ingredients: *Hyoscyamus niger* | Henbane

Throughout the general population seeds, capsules and leaves were smoked from this time to relieve toothache.

'In a monastery, where the roots of henbane had been eaten for supper, by mistake, those who partook of them were seized in the night with a curious kind of hallucination, and exhibited the most ridiculous antics, so that it was more like a lunatic asylum than a monastery; one rang the bell for matins at 12 o'clock at night; of the fraternity who attended to the summons, some could not read, some read what was not in the book; some saw the letters running about the page like ants.'

'It is related of a tailor that under the influence of this plant, he could not thread his needle, and that when his apprentice had threaded it for him, he could not hit the cloth but sometimes pricked his fingers and sometimes his thigh; his needle seemed to him to have three points. In old works there are many curious effects attributed to this herb'.

SHARP Practice Volume 4 1992 (Occasions of mild henbane poisoning reported in The Lancet, 1844).

Gustav Shenk experimented on himself in 1920 and wrote down his experience:

A number of henbane seeds were put on an iron plate before an open fire.

'The Henbane's, first effect was a purely physical discomfort. My limbs lost their certainty, pains hammered in my head and I began to feel extremely giddy. Fumes were still rising from the iron plate, so not much time can have elapsed before the onset of these initial symptoms, 15 minutes at most. I had the feeling that my head had increased in size; it seemed to have grown broader more solid and heavier.

I went to the mirror and was able to distinguish my face, but more dimly than normal; it looked flushed. The mirror itself was swaying and I found it difficult to keep my face within its frame. The black disc of my pupils were immensely enlarged as though the whole iris had become black. Despite the dilation of my pupils I could see no better than usual, quite the contrary, the outline of objects were hazy the windows and window frame were obscured by a thin mist.

To comprehend the power of black henbane, the reader must picture the following condition. The ears become deaf, the eyes almost blind; they see in a haze only the bulk of objects; whose contours are blurred. The sufferer is slowly cut off from the outside world and sinks irretrievably into himself and his own inner world.

Black henbane causes a general poisoning with symptoms of illness. The sense of being seriously ill does not leave one for an instant. The first inhalation of the fumes of the roasted seeds immediately arouses a feeling of extreme discomfort and general bodily weakness, which rises to a mingled enjoyment and terror accompanied by an unparalleled wealth of visual images, to which are added unknown sensations of smell and touch.'

Torquis infantum, a necklace for children

Cut pieces of male peony root and fresh henbane root and cut into round pieces, make a hole in the middle of each piece and thread on to a string. Wrap this in fine linen or lawn and place it around the neck of a teething infant. (*Certainly the effect of absorbing the juice from these roots into the child's blood stream would be quite powerful, certainly relaxing!*)

Conium maculatum | Hemlock

Apart from its use as a major ingredient in the medieval anaesthetic mixture hemlock has a well documented history as a poison.

399BC After his trial and conviction for impiety and corruption the Greek philosopher Socrates was sentenced to death by drinking a tea made from hemlock.

The most detailed observation of a more modern hemlock poisoning took place in Edinburgh in 1845:

"On the 21st April 1845 Duncan Gow, a 43 year old tailor was brought into the Royal Infirmary of Edinburgh by two police men. It was stated that he had been found lying in the street apparently in a state of intoxication or in a fit. On being taken into the waiting room, he was found to be dead."

According to the examining physician - John Huges Bennett, this case was the first 'minutely' detailed study of hemlock poisoning.

In his stomach were 11oz of some raw green vegetable resembling parsley.

Dr Christison, professor of materia medica was consulted and he pointed out that this vegetable material could scarcely be anything else than the laciniae of the conium maculatum or common hemlock. It smells mousy when bruised.

Duncan Gow evidently had had a palsy first of the voluntary muscles, next of the chest, lastly of the diaphragm followed by asphyxiation from paralysis without insensibility and with slight occasional twitches only of the limbs. The substantial intake of hemlock had led to his speedy death.

He ate bread and green salad, a favourite of his gathered by his children aged 10 and 6 for him from a bank under the Walter Scott Memorial. It was in the late afternoon and the man's first meal of the day.

They were not well off. From his home, at the head of Cannongate he had walked to West port - and sold goods there, his course unsteady and staggering.

Children taunted him "Get out of the way of the lame horse."

Policemen among others thought him drunk. He said that he had completely lost his sight, and had not the perfect use of his limbs. His legs bent under him and he fell upon his knees. A policeman then gave him some water to drink, which he was incapable of swallowing, and then helped him on to a barrow.

On lifting up his eyelids a police man found the eyes dull and his legs were trailing; he was now slowly carted to the main police office in the High Street. From the manner in which the man was lying, and from the loss of power in his legs, the police judged that he was not intoxicated. He was still able to give his address.

The police surgeon was sent for at 7.10 pm he reported all motion of the chest appeared to have ceased; the action of the heart was very feeble and the countenance had a cadaveric expression; his pupils were fixed. He was then sent to the infirmary and upon arrival he was dead. It was perhaps three hours since Duncan Gow ate hemlock.

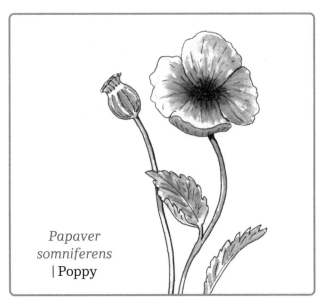

*Papaver
somniferens*
| Poppy

Papaver somniferum | **Poppy**

The history of Poppy medicine

Opium is derived from the latex produced by poppy seed heads which when scored produces exudate/latex which is refined into opium.

Opium doesn't impair sensory perception, the intellect or motor co-ordination. It eases pain and at lower doses opium may be pleasantly stimulating rather than soporific. Opium was probably the world's first anti depressant. It is habit forming and addictive.

The analgesics found in opium reduce pain without causing loss of consciousness, relieve coughs, spasms, fevers and diarrhoea.

• 28,000BC - Fossilised poppy seeds found in a Neanderthal grave.

• 4000BC - First written reference to opium in a Sumerian text as hul gil - plant of joy.

• 2000BC - Fossil remains of poppy-seed cake and poppy seed heads have been found in Neolithic lake-dwellings in Switzerland.

• C1 - Used widely in Greece - described by Galen in his writings - Greek Physicians ground up the whole plant or used opium extract. It was also popular in Egypt and is frequently represented on wall paintings.

• C8 - Opium use spreads to Arabia, India and China.

• C10 - A Chinese poem celebrates how the opium poppy can be made into a drink "fit for Buddha."

• Paracelsus (1490-1541) [Phiilippus Aureolus Theophrastus Bombastus von Hohenheim] known as the founder of chemical medicine said "I possess a secret remedy which I call laudanum and which is superior to all other heroic remedies". He extracted opium into brandy to create this new stronger remedy, a tincture of morphine. "The stone of immortality".

• C17 - Thomas Sydenham the 17th century pioneer of English medicine called opium "Among the remedies which it has pleased Almighty God to give to man to relieve his sufferings, none is so universal and so efficacious as opium". He also produced the first standardised laudanum formulation - 2oz opium, 1oz saffron, a drachm of cinnamon and cloves, all dissolved in a pint of Canary wine.

• C19 - Bottles of laudanum and raw opium were freely available at any English pharmacy or grocers. British imports increased from 91,000lbs in 1830 to 280,000lbs in 1860. Although Britain controlled Indian production most UK opium came from Turkey - due to a higher morphine content.

Samuel Taylor Coleridge (1772-1834) wrote the unfinished 'Kubla Khan' under the influence of opium.

Thomas De Quincey (1785-1859) wrote 'Confessions of an English Opium Eater' (1821).

Opium was De Quincey's 'Divine poppy-juice, as indispensable as breathing'.

The pharmacist C.R. Alder Wright in 1874 in an attempt to find a non addictive alternative to morphine boiled morphine with acetic acid to produce diacetylmorphine, which in 1898 was marketed by Bayer as heroin.

Youngsters were introduced to opiates in mill towns - baby minders used Godfrey's cordial, Street's Infant's Quietness, Atkinson's Infants' Preservative and Mrs Winslow's Soothing Syrup.

Extract from John Skelton Botanic record 1852
The Cotton Metropolis

"The greater number of Manchester's unnessary deaths are made up of children's deaths. It is before the juvenile portion of the population begin to work in the factory, not after it, that the system exposes them to the greatest danger. It is a melancholy, but undoubted fact, that out of every 100 deaths in Manchester, very nearly one half - 48 and a fraction - are those of children under five years of age; while placing the period of life at ten years, we find that 52 out of the 100 die annually. In some of the neighbouring towns, especially in Ashton-under-Lyne, the proportion is still more appalling. There, by a calculation made embracing the five years ending with June 1843, it appeared that out of the whole number of deaths, 57% were those of children under five years of age. It is of course generally known that the first five years of life are the most fatal in all districts; but the infant mortality of the cotton towns is nearly 20%, greater than the average of the whole kingdom. In this difference of proportion it is to be found the great evil of the factory system as it at present exists - an evil committed not directly by work at the mills, but indirectly by work at the mills drawing individuals in certain cases from their homes. Marriages in Manchester are frequently contracted at a very early age, long before the man has any chance of holding the better paid class of situations in the factory; and the result is, that his wife, like himself is obliged to continue her daily toil at the mill, even after she has a young family growing up around her. From this necessity comes the curse of the cotton towns - the dosing of the children with opium to keep them quietly asleep at home or at nurse, until the return of their mothers in the evening; and the fact, demonstrated by statistics, that every seven years 14,000 children die in Manchester over and above the natural proportions. As may be well supposed, the system of infant neglect continues even after the children have got too old to be left all day in the cradle. Then they wander forth into the streets, running the risk of all manner of accidents, and so frequently going astray, that the police have actually to find out the domiciles of upwards of 4000 'lost' children per annum. This fact is mentioned upon the authority of the constabulary returns annually made to the corporation.

'In Ashton-Under-Lyne' says a local medical authority, 'it is no infrequent occurrence for mothers of the tenderist age to return to their work in the factories on the second or third week after confinement, and to leave their helpless offspring in the care of mere girls and superannuated old women'. Sometimes a wet nurse is clubbed for by three or even four women. Mr Coultard has seen one so exhausted 'as to be unable to walk across the room' while the children

'were almost unable to move their hands or feet'. The wet-nurse however most frequently applied to is the laudanum bottle. The dose is sometimes administered by the mother before she leaves home, but more generally by the old women who are employed to take charge of perhaps half-a-dozen children, who are carried every morning to their house, and whom she doses so as to keep them quiet during the day, at a weekly stipend from 1s 6d to 2s 5d.

The effect of laudanum on the children is to produce a suffusion of the brain, and a whole tribe of glandular and mesenteric disorders. The child sinks into a low torpid state, and wastes away to a skeleton, the stomach alone preserving its protuberance. If it survives, it is more or less weakly, and stunted for life - the complexion never assumes a healthy hue, and the vital powers never attain their natural force and vigour. The liquid principally used is a drug common enough through all the country, and well known as 'Godfrey's cordial'. In Manchester, Godfrey as the term is generally abbreviated, is a household word.

The 'Godfrey' is an old fashioned preparation, and has been in use for nearly a century. It is made in different degrees of strength, but on the average contains about ounce and a half of laudanum to the quart. The dose is from half a teaspoonful to two teaspoonfuls. 'Infants Cordial' has the reputation of being stronger, containing on the average two ounces of laudanum to the quart. The stronger the potion is, indeed, the more it is sure to be in demand; and the dealers have a half empty bottle frequently brought to them, with a request for a drachm or so additional laudanum. The constituents of all these doses over and above the narcotic element are - water, aniseed, and treacle. The stuff is often made up wholesale in huge coppers holding as much as 20 gallons, and then supplied to the druggists and the general shops, to be frequently sold in the latter as 'children's draughts, a penny each'.

Sometimes the children are dosed by the nurse without the knowledge or consent of the mothers, who, however soon find out the truth by the languid air and wasting limbs of their offspring. But the administration of 'sleeping stuff', for the purpose of obtaining an undisturbed nights rest, is an almost universal practice even by parents who would shrink from stupefying their offspring in the daytime. Very young girls, too, when left in charge of children follow the usages of old nurses; and thus when every engine in Manchester is panting and throbbing, and every adult and youthful hand and eye upon the alert, a large proportion of the infant population is lying in a torpid sleep - their young engines sealed up , and their brains becoming softened under the spell of the wretched potion which has lulled them."

Claviceps purpurea | **Ergot**

Juniperus communis | **Juniper**

Ergot is a parasitic fungus growing out of the head of grasses and is frequently found on rye; during a talk given by Brian Moffat at the Soutra site he demonstrated that ergot continued to grow on grasses around Soutra Aisle up to the present day.

Alkaloids are produced by the Claviceps purperea fungus which appears as a black growth known as an ergot body.

Ergot flourishes on grain during damp conditions, for example a wet summer that produces a poor harvest. Bread made from ergot contaminated grain causes a condition called 'Holy Fire', currently known as gangrene.

Gangrene is the result of vasoconstriction induced by the ergotamine-ergocristine alkaloids of the fungus. Initially it affects fingers and toes. The vasoconstriction causes acute pain and the 'death' of the affected areas resulting in the loss of the digits. During this process gangrene sets in ultimately causing the death of the patient.

The Order of St. Anthony were particularly successful in treating ergot poisoning during the middle ages, ultimately giving the condition one of its names - St. Anthony's Fire. One of the first descriptions thought to be of 'Holy Fire' - 'Great plagues of swollen blisters consumed the people by a loathsome rot, so that their limbs were loosened and fell off before death'. Annales Xantenses 857 AD.

There is a useful side to ergot, it was used for many years in midwifery latterly under the name ergotamine, it is used in hospitals today to stop hemorrhaging. This effect was probably known in medieval times and the fact that it was found at Soutra with juniper, a powerful uterine stimulant, may indicate its therapeutic uses.

Childbirth can result in hemorrhaging - ergot stops bleeding, slow childbirth can be speeded up with a uterine stimulant - juniper has this effect.

Both these herbs are very powerful and alternatively may have been used as abortifacients.

Blood letting

'he bulk of the information from the excavations at outra comes from the drain that was linked to the nfirmary. On examination, he clay based soil that was found in the drain not only acted as an excellent medium for preserving rtefacts it was also full of a substance identified as olood. This was established definitively by using products available from GP surgeries for testing stool amples for traces of blood,(positive results forheam were found in trenches 1, 7 and 12) thus linking well with the fact that bloodletting in the middle ages was a standard part of monastic life.

There were rules to blood letting in medieval monasteries and here are a few guide lines that were laid down to ensure the comfort and safety of the blood letee.

Green Pharmacy - Barbara Griggs 1981

"Those who intend to be bled had to ask permission from the President in Chapter, having received their bleeding license from him they are to leave the Choir after the gospel at High Mass and go to the place to be bled - the infirmary. Two or three or four may be bled at the same time but no more or there may be too few left in the convent. During this time they ought not to enter the Choir for Matins or the other Hours, except on special occasions, such as processions, the presence of a corpse or at commendation on the anniversaries of Priors and the like.

"The period of bleeding lasted for three days. The master of the infirmary ought daily to provide a pittance (food), suitable to their condition and at fixed times with fire and a candle. Further, he is to provide a clean napkin and towels, goblets and spoons; and all utensils that they will require, and he ought to bestow on them all the comfort and kindness in his power, for those that have been bled ought during that period lead a life of joy and freedom from care, in comfort and happiness. Nor ought they in any way to annoy each other with sarcastic or abusive language. On this account they ought all to be careful to abstain from jeers and evil speaking, and also from games of dice and chess and other games unsuitable to those that lead a religious life because beyond all doubt, they are offensive to God and frequently give occasion to strife and contention among those who play them.

"No one therefore ought to do or say anything that can interfere with the comfort or the repose of those who have been bled. If, however, they take a fancy to walk through the vineyard or the garden to the other offices within the precincts, they are to ask leave of the Warden of the Order, but if they wish to go outside to take the air, they ought to ask leave of the Prelate himself, should he be at home."

In its heyday Soutra's precinct covered an area of forty acres thus proving a wide area in which to take the air.

Monks were encouraged to be bled approximately every seven weeks although some preferred to be bled more often; on these occasions they were expected to carry on with their normal routine within the monastery and not spend three days resting in the infirmary, possibly to prevent some from 'enjoying' the process.

Diet

On the first day of bleeding the servant of the infirmary ought at once to get ready for those who have been bled sage and parsley washed in water with salt in it, and, if times permit, soft eggs. On the second day those who have been bled ought not to celebrate Mass for fear they should chance to hurt the arm in which the vein has been opened.

On the third day they ought to enter the Chapter House and ask for pardon with their faces on the ground, and during the whole of that day stay in the infirmary for the continuance of their repose, but they ought to hasten into the Dorter to sleep there with the rest of the community.

What were the perceived benefits of bloodletting?

Bloodletting 'Clears the mind, strengthens the memory, cleanses the guts, dries up the brain, warms the marrow, sharpens the hearing, curbs tears, encourages discrimination, helps the stomach, develops the senses, promotes digestion, produces a musical voice, dispels sleepiness, drives away anxiety, feeds the blood, rids it of poisonous matter and gives a long life. It eliminates rheumatic ailments whilst getting rid of pestilent diseases, it cures pains, fevers and various sicknesses and makes urine clear and clean.'

It also lowers blood pressure, potentially a problem for the better fed monks.

Seyney Houses

The process would frequently take place in a warming room or special seyney room or house in the monastery precincts. The word 'seyney' is connected to the name 'Sinai' as in Sinai Park near Burton-Upon-Trent. The old house was used by the monks of Burton Abbey as a seyney house.

A History of Bloodletting

'A Latin Technical Phlebotomy' translated by Linda Voigts and Michael McVaughn.

This is a historical introduction to bloodletting in the Middle Ages and provides a summary of the key points. At Salerno in the late C11 and C12 there was a systematic reworking of Greco-Roman and earlier material on bloodletting; as the C12 progressed there was a gradual introduction of Arabic medical literature to the west, particularly the work of Constantine the African.

This work includes advice on how to ligature a limb to make the vein visible and how and in what direction to make the incision to avoid cutting a nerve. A lancet was used, a sharp blade in a variety of designs.

Constantine took the total of potential veins to use to five (previously there had been only three veins to choose from). There were contributions from Avicenna and Albucasis - both of whom had been translated from the Arabic by Gerard of Cremona. A comprehensive analysis of the practice of bloodletting had been established by the end of the C13.

Medical Practitioners and other Residents at Soutra

Only one medical practitioner figures in the Soutra archive. This is Master Martin the physician, although he does not appear in the directory of medical practitioners of medieval Britain whose records extend to 1518.

At its height Soutra had a resident religious community of about 30 souls plus servants, serfs and bondsmen - a large settlement which would equal the population of a small town and goes some way towards explaining the significant quantity of blood found in the drains.

Bacillus anthracis | Anthrax

The Medieval hospital at Soutra flourished from AD 1164 to 1462 and went into a progressive decline over the next 200 years.

There has been no occupancy of the Soutra hill top (1,100 feet) for the last 300 years but even if there had been some form of human presence on the site the deposits of infirmary waste containing large quantities of degraded blood including anthrax spores and herbal material, were safely sealed beneath a continuous layer of masonry and rubble. The clay matrix of the site is sterile, waterlogged and cold.

The anthrax spores were recovered from a soak-away at 1.2m beneath ground level and within the hospital living quarters. For this reason the spores are certainly human and not animal in origin.

There have been a number of isolated outbreaks of anthrax in cattle as recently as the 1940s and 1950s in the farms around Soutra. There have only been rare incidents of anthrax elsewhere in Scotland around this time making these events something of an anomaly, except that we know that it was present at Soutra during its occupation by the monastery as the presence of the endospores in the drains confirm. This is certainly an interesting coincidence.

Anthrax is an acute disease that is usually fatal, it is caused by the bacterium Bacillus anthracis. A distinguishing feature of the genus Bacillus is that in the form of endospores they are able to survive harsh conditions for centuries. When these spores are inhaled, ingested or come into contact with a skin lesion they may reactivate and multiply rapidly.

Until the C20 anthrax infections killed hundreds of thousands of animals and people worldwide each year, the first effective vaccine not being developed until Pasteur's breakthrough in 1881.

An anthrax infection may take several forms:

Pulmonary: this is caused by inhalation of anthrax spores and used to be known as 'woolsorters' or' ragpickers' disease. These people were more susceptible to the disease owing to their exposure to infected animal products. Other vulnerable workers included those who sliced up animal horns to make buttons, or those who handled animal skins or hair bristles used to make brushes. This is the most common and fatal type of infection often resulting in pneumonia.

Gastrointestinal: acute inflammation of the intestinal tract caused by eating infected meat. Rare but often fatal causing vomiting of blood.

Cutaneous/skin: causes a painless necrotic ulcer which is not usually fatal.

Extracts

Extract from John Skelton
Botanic record 1852

John Skelton (1805 - 1880) was a Chartist and a Socialist as a young man and he kept to these principles throughout his life. In 1848 he became a herbalist, practising using Thompsonian principles (principles according to Samuel Thompson an American herbalist). Despite his training eriving from America he predominately used British herbs referring to early English herbalists Gerard and Parkinson among others. He believed that encouraging working class people to study Botanic Medicine - iving them some control over their own health - was empowering for people who had little control over their lives.

From James Searton - Carrier, New Brinsley, Nottingham. May 1852

"My symptoms were - difficulty in breathing, being unable to lie down either night or day, and a violent cough, accompanied by expectoration of purulent bloody matter - up to a pint a day, with blood gushing from the nose. After trying all the ways I could think or hear of to get better and getting worse daily , until I was so ill many of my friends had said goodbye to me expecting my children to be fatherless and my wife a widow very soon.

"When I heard how successful your botanic agent Mr Boot had been in arresting and curing this terrible disease.

"I had an appointment with him on 11th November 1849 , after taking the medicine for one week my appetite returned, my breathing eased so that I could lie down and by 24th December 1849 I was so recovered that I could go back to work much to everyone's amazement, and I have remained in good health ever since."

The treatment was as follows according to Mr Boot;
Horehound, centaury, ground ivy, raspberry leaves, clivers, agrimony, barberry bark, elecampane, marshmallow root, ginger. 1 oz of each of the above herbs boiled in three pints of water reduced to 1 1/2 pints taken by the wineglass full 4 times daily plus a teaspoonful of the cough syrup - liquorice juice 1/4 oz, bitter almonds 1/4 oz - three times daily.

Diagnosis
The amount of blood and pus produced daily by James Stearton plus his miraculous recovery indicates that he was probably suffering from empyema - 'pus in a body cavity especially in the pleural cavity usually the result of a primary infection in the lungs.' *Taber's Cyclopedic Medical Dictionary*. (These days this condition would be treated by drainage of the affected area and the use of antibiotics)

Symptoms of Empyema
Chills, fever, facial flushing, poor appetite, extreme tiredness, pain in chest, cough and emaciation (dramatic weight loss), difficulty in breathing.

Looking in a more detailed way at the herbs mentioned by Mr Boot the botanic agent, from Macer's perspective and in current C21 usage

Many of these herbs are found in Macer, some are in the later additions referred to in Ludwig Choulant's translation in 1832 as well as editions by Cornarius and Ranzowius.

White horehound / *Marubium vulgare* [Macer 53]:
Macer: primarily for coughs, when drunk in wine it 'destroys all poisons' bacterial infections? Fever and catarrh.
Current uses: expectorant, soothes coughs and is a tonic, acute bronchitis, whooping cough.

Centaury / *Centaurium erythraea* [Macer 42]:
Macer: primarily cooling, known as a 'fever chaser' also very healing to damaged tissue, stops bleeding.
Current uses: cooling, mild sedative, bitter tonic, antiinflammatory.

Ground ivy / *Glechoma hederacea* [later edition of Macer]:
Current uses: cooling, tonic, anti inflammatory, all types of catarrh - bronchial, nasal, deafness due to catarrh, tonic to mucus membranes.

Raspberry leaves / *Rubus iaedias* [later edition of Macer]:
Current uses: sooths spasms, astringent tonic, stops bleeding.

Clivers / *Galium aperine*:
Current uses: in common use - detoxifier, cooling, anti inflammatory, cleansing.

Agrimony / *Agrimonia europea*:
Current uses: in common use mild astringent, healing, bitter tonic, tonic to a sluggish liver, promotes assimilation of food.

Barberry bark / *Berberis vulgaris*:
Current uses: in common use as a liver stimulant, a tonic for the spleen and pancreas, as a mild sedative, antihaemorrhagic, antibacterial.

Elecampane / *Inula helenium* [Macer 18]:
Macer: helps with coughs and aids breathing.
Current uses: to soothe acute bronchitis, brochiectasis, asthma, coughs.

Marshmallow root / *Althea radix* [Macer 66]
Macer: soothing, very healing to all parts of the body, heals bleeding wounds.
Current uses: soothing, reduces inflammation, soothes asthma symptoms and those of acute or chronic bronchitis.

Ginger / *Zingiber officinale* [Macer 69]
Macer: similar to pepper; helps improve the efficiency of digestion and eases discomfort in the stomach, cooling.
Current uses: improves circulation, reduces inflammation, is a digestive,soothes acute bronchitis, fevers and common cold, asthma.

Liquorice / *Glycyrriza glabra* [Macer 86]
Macer: primarily for bringing up phlegm and moistening sick lungs, for a harsh cough and the ease of congestion of the chest.
Current uses: anti inflammatory, expectorant, soothes coughs, acute or chronic bronchitis, used to soothe gastro-oesophageal reflux.

Bitter almonds:
Current uses: digestive tonic and a source of protein.

Sources:
Macer, Encyclopaedia
of Herbal Medicine
by Thomas Bartram,
The Ultimate Herbal
Compendium
by Kerry Bone.

Soutra and Macer: a summary of health care

Although Macer comments on herbal remedies that may have been beneficial treatments, the use of any of this information as a treatment of any kind is at the readers own risk.

We know that the monastery at Soutra was established about the same time that the book Macer Floridus De Viribus Herbarium was written. The book mainly used information from books written by Dioscorides and Pliny the Elder, from these writings a compact pocket sized book evolved - covering all illnesses - serious and minor, that might crop up in daily life. Alongside the original information about the plants there are additional comments made by the author which give practical guidance on how to use and prepare the herbs; and under which conditions to use specific herbs including the recommended dosages. This was essential information for physicians - who were able to read Latin - and who were largely to be found in monastic foundations.

Many of the names of the illnesses are surprisingly familiar to a modern reader as the derivation of these names is from Latin. i.e. sciatica, gout, cirrhosis, jaundice, parotids.

It was clearly not written from a Northern European perspective, although many of the herbs are familiar some cannot be found in such an unpredictable climate. In fact, at least on two occasions, herbs such as myrtle and spikenard are mentioned with an additional reference to the Celtic or Northern variety - indicating that these herbs could be used in a similar fashion to the Middle Eastern or Greek species.

We, in the 21st century, have the impression that medicine in the middle ages was a primitive affair relying more on superstition, charms and witch craft than medicine as we understand it. This may have been true in some instances as there are mentions of using herbs as charms to ward off death by drowning, wild dogs or being bitten by venomous beasts.

Apart from these instances Macer was pragmatic and the remedies offered may well have been effective in achieving relief from symptoms or even cures, although it has to be imagined that the use of some of the more toxic plants may have led to death rather than recovery.

Looking at the most common conditions mentioned in Macer

Women's complaints

Particularly notable is the delivery of a deformed child or 'warpling'. Pennyroyal is specifically mentioned with reference to initiating the delivery of a 'warpling', but we can only speculate as to how they would have known of its deformity. Pennyroyal can also bring on a delayed period or induce a miscarriage. The complete elimination of the afterbirth was an area that was also covered very thoroughly with a wide selection of herbs suggested to facilitate this. If this wasn't achieved the mother would die due to infection and until the discovery of antibiotics all elements of child birth were fraught with danger to both mother and child.

Heavy periods - there are many herbs mentioned in Macer that could be taken to ease menorrhagia.

Contraception - something that may be considered to have been beyond people 1000 years ago - mint leaves placed in the cervix or aniseed tea - drunk frequently are the two methods mentioned in Macer (the efficacy of these herbal forms of contraception is unconfirmed).

Swellings and infections of the womb are all addressed by more herbs than any other area of the body. Many monks were in closed orders which did not include women but in the case of Soutra and other Augustinian monasteries medical treatment was available to everyone; Macer was clearly written for the use of educated people with an interest in medicine, including monks.

Digestive illnesses

Poor digestion, stomach issues and liver problems are also considered in detail - some of the herbs in this section are used by herbalists today and in many cases for similar conditions. Frequently mentioned are issues with the spleen - splenic conditions are only treated occasionally by modern herbalists, this may be due to a difference in the perception of the underlying cause.

Vermifuges or treatments for parasites and worms are also frequently mentioned (often not just in relation to the digestive system, they sometimes refer to worms in the womb, ear or teeth - this might have been a way of describing the 'sensation' rather than worms actually being found in these areas). Wormwood/ Artemisia absinth is a classic herb for killing intestinal worms and continues to be used today. In the middle ages parasite infestations were very common and therefore regular courses of wormwood or similar were taken to control the infestation. In Scotland they used finely ground Tormentil root- a locally available herb - mixed into porridge - this mixture was found in the drains at Soutra. These days there is less familiarity with parasites and worms but even today they are thought to be potentially the underlying cause of a variety of chronic conditions.

The 'bloody flux' was a constant risk and required fast efficient treatment - the possibility of dying very quickly from dehydration or blood loss was a genuine risk. Also there seems to have been quite a variety of fevers that could occur for unknown reasons - but each was observed and given a name as well as a specific treatment.

Kidney and bladder stones

These were apparently as common a thousand years ago as they were in the 1600s when Samuel Pepys had the stone in his bladder removed - without anaesthetic. At Soutra there would have been the option of using an anaesthetic. These days we recognise that kidney and bladder stones develop if someone eats an acidic diet, high in protein with little fruit, vegetables or water. Although today people do suffer from kidney stones it was a much more common complaint historically. Preferred drinks were a variety
of wines which are acid forming and would contribute to the formation of kidney and bladder stones as well as gout - apparently another common condition. Beer was more available in England and Scotland - where heather beer was brewed. This was a time when the cleanliness of drinking water was uncertain and converting it into a form of alcohol provided some protection from water borne diseases.

Although not mentioned in Macer - the henbane, hemlock and opium blend that was found in the drains at Soutra was used as a very effective, if potentially lethal, anaesthetic - this mixture or variations on these herbs are found in various texts written in the Middle Ages.

Wounds

There are references to arrow and spear wounds in Macer and wild arach or clematis if made into a plaster could be used to draw out 'nails or spears'. To heal a wound - Herb Bennet (Geum urbanum) will 'cleanse a wound and afterwards fill it with good flesh'. These were times of war throughout Europe. At Soutra, war wounds would have been common - the border between England and Scotland was continually shifting throughout Soutra's existence. There were frequent battles locally - Bannockburn is within sight of Soutra. Other wounds were probably due to domestic or industrial injury.

Emotional trauma

Living in a war zone has a damaging effect emotionally on people and this is clearly the case at Soutra. Finding the remains of Valerian (Valeriana officianalis) and St. Johns wort (Hypericum perforatum) in the drains mixed together suggests that a calming and uplifting drink was required at times. Hypericum is well documented as an anti-depressant which is used effectively today; it is not mentioned in Macer and Valerian is only mentioned briefly for the treatment of fevers, currently it is often used for its calming effect on the nervous system, the effect is almost instant and doesn't cause drowsiness. Clearly, although Macer was the main medical reference book, it was not used exclusively and local herbal knowledge was also sought and applied. Other uplifting herbs mentioned in Macer are - Sweet Cyprus - if drunk as a tea, will have a calming and uplifting effect on the spirits Italian Bugloss has a cheering and uplifting effect when taken as a drink, it also improves the memory. Rue juice if blended with an equal quantity of Elecampane juice and infused together makes 'a valuable medicine if it is drunk by people who have been 'broken'', (the exact meaning of this statement is unclear, it may refer to emotional breakdown).

Peony has a reputation for preventing nightmares and if the root is boiled and eaten by a lunatic - they will be healed. Lettuce seed tea, it is suggested, will prevent frightening dreams - as it is a soporific it would potentially allow the patient to sleep through their nightmares.

Headaches, coughs, chest conditions and eyesight problems

These were fairly common and were probably a result of living in smoky conditions. Many people lived in one or two rooms with an open hearth for cooking and a hole in the roof to let the smoke out.

Holy Fire or ergot poisoning

This has already been mentioned and is very rare now - the fungus affects damp grain, in times of a poor harvest the temptation to eat or sell this grain may have been overwhelming. Although the nerve damage and pain associated with it (often depicted as flames coming out of the hands or feet, indicating the level and type of pain involved) would have been hard to treat; using rose oil and poppy juice would have provided some relief.

Beauty aids of the Middle Ages

There has been significant interest in looking beautiful throughout history. Many of the herbs mentioned are for removing unsightly blemishes from the face.

Other areas of concern were:

Wrinkles - lily roots if ground up with creote or wax and butter and applied to the face - may smooth out wrinkles and eliminate freckles if used regularly.

Baldness - watercress, onion juice or cabbage blended with alum and sharp vinegar and applied to the head will encourage hair regrowth.

Dandruff - violet juice rubbed onto the head will cure this.

Grey hair - sage juice will make grey hair black if applied in the heat of the sun.

Freckles - white or black pepper, celery juice, or onion mixed with vinegar and if applied to the face will remove them. Some of these remedies would probably have replaced the freckle with a scar -perhaps not a satisfactory exchange e.g. take two parts powdered iris root and one part powdered hellebore root and blend together with honey - apply to the freckles, pockets or welks on the face. A potent mixture.

In conclusion   The drains at Soutra have provided a fascinating glimpse of what life in a busy monastery on a major route between two warring countries might have been like between 1150 AD and 1420 AD. Perhaps more advanced than we might imagine, they were certainly creative in the use of plants and other materials available at the time to try to maintain good health. As we now realise many 'old wives tales' are based on sound logic and observation with current scientific research backing up some of these ideas.

Index of herbs
Latin name

Allium ampeloprasum 11 (page 22)

Allium cepa 26 (page 52)

Allium sativum 5 (page 10)

Aloe vulgaris 78 (page 136)

Alpinia officianale 71 (page 128)

Althea officianalis 66 (page 119)

Althea Rosea 22 (page 42)

Anchusa italica/atrigosa 51 (page 92)

Anthriscus cerefolium 36 (page 69)

Apium graviolens 9 (page 19)

Aristolochia clematis 8 (page 17)

Artemisia abrotanum 2 (page 5)

Artemisia absinth 3 (page 6)

Artemisia vulgaris 1 (page 4)

Asarum europeum
54/102 (page 97/162)

Atriplex patula 33 (page 64)

Atropa mandragora page XXVIII

Basillus anthracis page LIX

Beta vulgaris 82 (page 142)

Boswellia sacra 77 (page 135)

Brassica 25 (page 49)

Brassica nigra/Sinapsis alba
27 (page 54)

Brionia dioica 97 (page 157)

Calendula officinalis 83 (page 143)

Carum carvi 90 (page 150)

Centaurium erythraea 42 (page 79)

Cheledonium majus
| Ranunculus ficaria 59 (page107)

Cinnamomum verum 74 (page 131)

Claviceps purpurea page LV

Conium maculatum
39 (page 74/XLIX)

Coriandrum sativum 32 (page 62)

Costus arabicus 75 (page 132)

Crocus sativum 89 (page 149)

Cuminium cyminum 70 (page 127)

Curcuma longa 72 (page 129)

Cyperus articulatus 55 (page 99)

Datura stramonium 105 (page 165)

Dracunculus vulgaris 44 (page 81)

Foeniculum vulgare 13 (page 26)

Gentian amarelle 81 (page 141)

Geum urbanum 92 (page 152)

Glycyrrhiza glabra 86 (page 146)

Gonecera periclinenum
| Levisticum officinale 46 (page 85)

Helleborus alba 61 (page 109)

Helleborus niger 62 (page 112)

Hyoscyamus niger
65 (page 117/XLVIII)

Hyssopus officinalis 20 (page 38)

Inula helenium 18 (page 35)

Iris germanic 21 (page 40)

Isatis tictora 60 (page 108)

Juniperus communis 10 (page 21)

Lactuca virosa 14 (page 28)

Laurus noblis 85 (page 145)

Levisticum officinale | Gonecera
periclinenum 46 (page 85)

Lilium album 16 (page 31)

Lupinus alba 104 (page 164)

Marubium vulgare 53 (page 95)

Matricaria recutita 45 (page 83)

Melissa officialis 57 (page 103)

Mentha longifolia 95 (page 155)

Mentha piperita 34 (page 65)

Mentha pulegium 40 (page 76)

Myristica fragrans 87 (page 147)

Myrtus communis 88 (page 148)

Nardostachys jatamans 76 (page 133)

Nasturtium officianale 29 (page 57)

Nepeta cataria 12 (page 24)

Nigella sativa 38/101 (page 73/161)

Oreganum dictamnus 93 (page153)

Orobus silvaticus page XLIV

Paeonia officinale 56 (page 101)

Papaver somniferen 31 (page 60/LI)

Parietaria officinalis 68 (page 124)

Pastinacea sativa 35 (page 67)

Pimpinella anisum 23 (page 44)

Pimpernella saxifrage 80 (page 140)

Pimpinella saxifraga 91 (page 151)

Piper album 28 (page 56)

Piper nigrum 67 (page 122)

Plantago major/lanceolata 6 (page 12)

Portulaca oleracea 49 (page 89)

Puliole haunt 52 (page 93)

Raphanus sativus 98 (page 158)

Ranunculus ficaria
| Cheledonium majus 59 (page 107)

Rosa canina 15 (page 29)

Rumex acetosa 47 (page 86)

Rumex acetosella 48 (page 88)

Rumex patiens 37 (page 71)

Ruta graviolens 7 (page 15)

Salvia officinalis 19 (page 37)

Salvia sclarea 100 (page 160)

Sanicula europa 79 (page 139)

Saponaria officinalis 50 (page 90)

Satureja hortensis 17 (page 33)

Scrophularia nodosa 96 (page 156)

Senecio vulgaris 58 (page 105)

Sinapsis alba | Brassica nigra
27 (page 54)

Solanum nigrum 64 (page 116)

Stachys betonica 24 (page 46)

Syzygium aromaticum 73 (page 130)

Tanacetum parthenium 94 (page 154)

Tanacetum vulgaris 84 (page 144)

Teucrium chamaedrys 43 (page 80)

Thymus vulgaris 41 (page 78)

Trigonella foenumgraecum
99 (page 159)

Urtica dioica 4 (page 8)

Valeriana officinalis 103 (page 163)

Verbena officinalis 63 (page 114)

Viola odorata 30 (page 58)

Zingiber officinale 69 (page 126)

Index of herbs
Medieval
name

Althea | Hocke 66 (page 119)

Anyse 23 (page 44)

Arage | Arach 33 (page 64)

Baldmoyne 81 (page 141)

Balm 57 (page 103)

Bawme 95 (page 155)

Beta 82 (page 142)

Betoyne 24 (page 46)

Black Ellebore 62 (page 112)

Brother Wort | Pyloile 40 (page 76)

Bysshopswort 50 (page 90)

Canel 74 (page 131)

Carmele | Carameile
   | Heath pea page XLIV

Celydone 59 (page 107)

Centory 42 (page 79)

Cerfoile 36 (page 60)

Chamomille 45 (page 83)

Clowe gelofre 73 (page 130)

Comyn 70 (page 127)

Coriundre 32 (page 62)

Coste 75 (page 132)

Coul 25 (page 49)

Cyperus 55 (page 99)

Ditayne 93 (page 153)

Dokke 37 (page 71)

Dragance 44 (page 81)

Featherfoy 94 (page 154)

Frankensence 77 (page 135)

Gamodreos 43 (page 80)

Garlik 5 (page 10)

Gladene 21 (page 40)

Groundswely 58 (page 105)

Gwade 60 (page 108)

Gyngyrere 69 (page 126)

Hocke | Althea 66 (page 119)

Horhoune 53 (page 95)

Horsehelene 18 (page 35)

Isope 20 (page 38)

Iubarbe 48 (page 88)

Kockul 38 (page 73)

Langedboef 51 (page 92)

Laureole 85 (page 145)

Leeke 11 (page 22)

Lupinus 104 (page 164)

Mandragora page XXVIII

Mille-Morbia 96 (page 156)

Mirtus 88 (page 148)

Morell 64 (page 116)

Mynte 34 (page 65)

Nasturtium 29 (page 57)

Nepe 97 (page 157)

Nepis 12 (page 24)

Notemuge 87 (page 147)

Oynones 26 (page 52)

Peletre 68 (page 124)

Persile 41 (page 78)

Planteyn 6 (page 12)

Pyloile | Brother Wort 40 (page 76)

Pympernolle 80 (page 140)

Pyoney 56 (page 101)

Raddish 98 (page 158)

Rewe 7 (page 15)

Rhodewort 83 (page 143)

Safron 89 (page 149)

Sanuerye 17 (page 33)

Satan's Apple page XXVIII

Saueyne 10 (page 21)

Saxifrage 91 (page 151)

Sclareye 100 (page 160)

Senueye 27 (page 54)

Smalache 9 (page 19)

Smerewort 8 (page 17)

Softe 54 (page 97)

Sorell 47 (page 86)

Verveyn 63 (page 114)

Vyldmalwe 22 (page 42)

White Ellebore 61 (page 109)

Wodebynd 46 (page 85)

Zeduale 72 (page 129)

Index of herbs
Common name

Aloe 78 (page 136)
Aniseed 23 (page 44)
Anthrax page LIX
Azara 102 (page 162)
Beet 82 (page 142)
Bennet 92 (page 152)
Bitter Vetch page XLVI
Black Hellebore 62 (page 112)
Black Nightshade 64 (page 116)
Bryony 97 (page 157)
Cabbage 25 (page 49)
Caraway 90 (page 150)
Catmint 12 (page 24)
Celandine Greater/Lesser
  59 (page 107)
Celery 9 (page 19)
Centaury 42 (page 79)
Chamomile 45 (page 83)
Chervil 36 (page 69)
Cinnamon 74 (page 131)
Clary Sage 100 (page 160)
Clematis 8 (page 17)
Clove 73 (page 130)
Coriander 32 (page 62)
Cumin 70 (page 127)
Dittany 93 (page 153)
Dock 37 (page 71)
Dragonwort 44 (page 81)
Elecampane 18 (page 35)
Ergot page LV
European Ginger 54 (page 97)

Fennel 13 (page 26)
Fenugreek 99 (page 159)
Feverfew 94 (page 154)
Figwort 96 (page 156)
Frankincense 77 (page 135)
Galingale 71 (page 128)
Garlic 5 (page 10)
Gentian 81 (page 141)
Germander 43 (page 80)
Ginger 69 (page 126)
Git 101 (page 161)
Groundsel 58 (page 105)
Hemlock 39 (page 74/XLIX)
Henbane 65 (page 117)
Hollyhock 22 (page 42)
Horehound 53 (page 95)
Horsemint 95 (page 155)
Hyssop 20 (page 38)
Iris 21 (page 40)
Italian Bugloss 51 (page 92)
Juniper 10 (page 21/LV)
Laurel 85 (page 145)
Leek 11 (page 22)
Lemon Balm 57 (page 103)
Lesser Wild Arach 33 (page 64)
Lesser Burnet 91 (page 151)
Lettuce 14 (page 28)
Lily 16 (page 31)
Liquorice 86 (page146)
Lovage 46 (page 85)
Lupin 104 (page 164)
Mandrake page XXVIII
Marigold 83 (page 143)
Marshmallow 66 (page 119)
Mint 34 (page 65)
Mugwort 1 (page 4)
Mustard 27 (page 54)
Myrtle 88 (page 148)
Bennet 92 (page 152)
Nettle 4 (page 8)
Nigella 38 (page 73)

Nutmeg 87 (page 147)
Of the Ginger Family 75 (page 132)
Onions 26 (page 52)
Oregano 52 (page 93)
Pellitory of the Wall 68 (page 124)
Pennyroyal 40 (page 76)
Peony 56 (page 101)
Pepper 67 (page 122)
Pimpernel 80 (page 140)
Plantain/Ribwort 6 (page 12)
Poppy 31 (page 60/LI)
Purslane 49 (page 89)
Radish 98 (page 158)
Ribwort 6 (page 12)
Rose 15 (page 29)
Rue 7 (page 15)
Sage 19 (page 37)
Saffron 89 (page 149)
Sanicle 79 (page 139)
Savory 17 (page 33)
Sheep Sorrel 48 (page 88)
Skyrwhit 35 (page 67)
Soapwort 50 (page 90)
Sorrel 47 (page 86)
Southernwood 2 (page 5)
Spikenard 76 (page 133)
Sweet Cyprus 55 (page 99)
Tansy 84 (page 144)
Thorn Apple 105 (page 165)
Thyme 41 (page 78)
Tumeric 72 (page 129)
Valerian 103 (page 163)
Vervane 63 (page 114)
Violet 30 (page 58)
Watercress 29 (page 57)
White Hellebore 61 (page 109)
White Pepper 28 (page 56)
Wode 60 (page 108)
Wood Betony 24 (page 46)
Wormwood 3 (page 6)

Glossary

A

Ache of the bladder - cystitis.

Adrenal restorative – restores/heals depleted adrenal glands.

Ague - a fever involving shivering and a high temperature.

Anointed – herbal preparation applied externally to areas of the body.

Antiallergic – reduces allergic responses to allergy triggers.

Antibacterial – active against bacteria.

Anticatarrhal – prevents the accumulation of mucous – usually in the respiratory system.

Antihaemorrhagic – stops heavy bleeding.

Anti-inflammatory – reduces inflammation.

Antirheumatic – eases the pain and inflammation of rheumatism.

Antispasmodic – relaxes and soothes spasms in smooth muscle.

Antitussive - a medicine or herb which eases a cough by reducing the cough reflex. A cough suppressant.

Antiulcer – heals ulcerated areas.

Antiviral – against viruses.

Analgesic - pain relieving.

Anxiolytic - medication which inhibits anxiety.

Asphyxiation – suffocation.

B

Brayed - pounded or crushed into small pieces typically in a pestle and mortar.

C

Cephalargia - headache.

Chink/chincough/chincost - whooping cough.

Creeping swellings - the exact meaning of this in the text is unclear. It could refer to 'creeping myiasis' which occurs when parasitic maggots penetrate the human skin most commonly in such exposed areas as the extremities, the back and the scalp. The unfortunate victim serves as an accidental host for these insects which could include several species of hypoderma. The primary symptom is a painful swelling that 'creeps' throughout the body as the larvae migrate and look for suitable sites for development.

Ciatus - the quantity 1/2 an egg shell can hold.

Creosote/create (sic) - a substance formed by the long ago distillation of various tars and by pyrolysis of plant derived material such as wood or fossil fuel. Used as an antiseptic or preservative.

D

Decoction - the simmering of woody material in water - root or bark - to extract the active constituents so that they may be taken by the patient as a medicine.

Diagredium - an ingredient in a laxative mixture.

Diuretic - a herb or medicine that promotes urination.

Dropsy - fluid retention in the body and limbs due to heart failure.

Demulcent - a substance which soothes irritation of for example, the mucous membrane.

Dragme - Medieval Latin form of the word 'dram' or 'drachm'. This was a unit of weight formerly used by apothecaries. It was the equivalent to 60 grains or 1/8 of an ounce. It could also be a liquid measure equivalent to 60 minims or 1/8 of a fluid ounce.

Dysentery – infection of the intestines resulting in severe diarrhoea.

E

Empicos - asthma.

Empyema - a collection of pus in the cavity of the pleura (the area which surrounds the lung).

Enema - a procedure in which liquid is introduced into the rectum as a means of administering a medicine or to expel the contents of the rectum.

Exudate - a mass of cells and fluid which has seeped out of blood vessels or an organ owing to inflammation.

Expectorant - medicine which increases the secretion of sputum through the airways. Used to relieve mucous congestion in chest infections by making coughs 'productive'.

F

Falling evil/falling sickness - epilepsy.

Flux / bloody flux - diarrhoea containing blood.

Febrifuge - literally a fever-chaser. A medicine which reduces fever.

Frankincense - an aromatic gum

resin obtained from trees of the genus Boswellia.

Fistula – an abnormal passage between a tubular organ, e.g. the intestines and the body surface. It can be caused by injury, surgery or from an infection or inflammation.

G

Gangrene – localised death and decomposition of body tissue by an anaerobic bacterium.

Genus bacillus – taxomic category ranking above species and below family referring to a specific bacterium.

Gastric bleeding – bleeding from the digestive system usually the stomach.

Gletty - green, slimy, oily.

Gobbettes - disc shaped slices cut from a plant or root.

Grain – a medieval weight, the smallest unit of weight in the troy and avoirdupois systems.

H

Humours / doctrine of humours - This doctrine is derived from the Greek physician Hippocrates (c460 - c370 BC). He incorporated the four temperaments into his medical theories:

Sanguine - social and enthusiastic,
Choleric - quick tempered and irritable,
Phlegmatic - easy going and peaceful,
Melancholic - quiet, sad and wise.

He believed that these four bodily fluids affected human behaviour as they moved around the body. His idea has since been discredited.

Holy Fire - ergot poisoning. In the medieval period the form of

poisoning caused by a species of fungus on rye or other cereals was known as St Anthony's Fire, named after monks of the Order of St Anthony who treated this ailment successfully. The name 'Holy Fire' described the nature of the pain experienced by sufferers.

In 1976 Linda Caporael suggested that the Salem witch trials followed an outbreak of ergot poisoning. The poison would, she claimed, have been sufficient to produce hallucinations among the victims which could have been interpreted as Satanic possession.

Haemoptysis - coughing up blood from the respiratory tract.

Hypotensive – reduces blood pressure.

I

Infusion - a drink, remedy or an extract prepared by soaking/infusing parts of a plant in a liquid.

Ingested – eaten.

J

K

Kernells - morbid formations of a rounded form occurring in the body, especially in enlarged lymph glands in the neck or groin.

Kerson - cardamon.

L

Latex - a milky fluid found in plants.

Laxative - a medicine which stimulates the emptying of the bowels.

Lesion - tissue damage - wound, ulcer, abscess or tumour.

Lichene - measles.

Litharge - lead monoxide, especia red form used as a pigment.

M

Materia medica - healing materi used to describe books compiled o information about healing plants.

Matrix - a mass of fine grained ro

Mulsa - a drink made of 8 parts w and one part honey.

Mula - chilblains.

Myrrh - an aromatic gum resin w flows from a tree resembling the acacia found in Arabia and Africa. is known as Balsamodendron myr to botanists.

N

Narcotic - an addictive drug inducing stupor or insensibility an also relieving pain.

Nervine - a medicine used to calm the nerves. Nervine herbs include skullcap, valerian, hops and chamomile.

Nitrum - also 'nitre'. Known historically as Nitrum Flammans, (chem.), probably so called because deflagrates when suddenly heated Ammonium Nitrate.

O

Oxymel - a drink made from 2 par vinegar to 3 parts honey.

Orthonoyci - archaic word for a t of asthma in which the patient is o able to breathe when upright.

Obulus - a medieval measure equa a scripulus.

P

Parocida - a pustule that develop the salivary gland.

Pastinaca - parsnip.

Periodica febris - fevers that occur periodically.

Peripheral vasodilator - dilates the blood vessels to the extremeties.

Pessary - a small soluble block inserted into the vagina to treat infection or as a contraceptive.

Pleura - each of a pair of membranes lining the thorax and enveloping the lungs in humans and other mammals.

Potage - a thick soup usually containing herbs. From the French.

Potager garden - a French term for an ornamental vegetable or kitchen garden.

Poultice - a soft, usually warm and sometimes medicated, mass spread on a cloth and applied to sores, wounds or lesions to relieve pain, supply warmth, to draw out pus/matter or to act as a counter-irritant or antiseptic.

Preterm foetus - birth occurring after a pregnancy significantly shorter than the normal 40 weeks.

Purgative - strongly laxative in effect.

Pusca - a drink made of one part vinegar and two parts water.

Pyment - wine infused with honey and spices.

Q

Quartan fever - a fever which reoccurs every 72 hours.

Quotidian fever - a fever which reoccurs every day.

Quinsy/quinsies - a suppurating infection of the tonsils.

R

S

Sapa - hot wine mixed with the juice of a herb.

Scabies - also called the 'itch mite'. The pregnant female burrows under the skin causing intense itching.

Scammony - a plant of the convolvulus family; the dried roots of the plant yield a strong purgative.

Scripulus - a medieval measure equal to an obulus.

Scrofula - this is the old term used for lymphadenopathy which is usually a result of either a tubercular or non-tubercular bacterial infection of the lymph nodes of the neck. Scrofula has been known since antiquity; during the Middle Ages the King's touch was believed to cure the disease - a belief which continued until the reign of Queen Anne.

Scruple - an old unit of weight equal to 20 grains; used by apothecaries.

Sedative - a preparation that encourages sleep.

Seethe - of a liquid - to boil.

Serplgo - a creeping spreading skin disease such as ringworm.

Soporific - inducing sleep.

Steep - to soak in water or any other fluid so as to soften, cleanse or extract some constituent from, say, a plant.

Styptic - a substance capable of causing bleeding to stop when it is applied to a wound.

Styptic - stops light bleeding.

Spasmolytic - a substance able to relieve muscle spasms.

Subluxation - partial dislocation of a joint.

Suppurate - the formation of pus in an injury owing to infection.

T

Tensamon - continual desire to empty the contents of the bowels or the bladder.

Tertian fever - a fever which reoccurs at 48 hour intervals.

Thymoleptic - uplifting.

The scab - scabies.

U

Uterus - womb.

V

Variole - measles.

Virum passum - a wine which has been squeezed out of dry grapes dried in the sun i.e. raisins.

Vermifuge - a medicine which causes the death or expulsion of intestinal worms e.g. tapeworms. Literally worm chasers.

Vulnery herbs - herbs which bring about healing in wounds either as skin lesions (emollients) or for internal wounds e.g. ulcers (demulcents).

W

Whirlbone - hip.

Wherpling/warpling - deformed child.

Welks - blemishes.

Wen - a boil or some other form of growth on the skin, especially used to refer to sebaceous cysts.

X

Y

Z

Zerna - (obsure) leprosy scar.

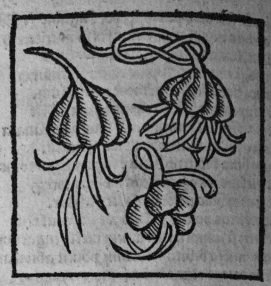

De voce ⁊ vmibꝫ.

De vmib⁹ ⁊ tineis

de morſu peſtifero.
De dolore veſice.

De ſcdis emiſſis
poſt partum
De pulmone.

De ydropicis.
De neuſreticis.

De yctericis.

De ventre duro.
De capitis dolore.

Et vocen̄/vermes/ſolo pelluntur odore
In mulſa coctum̄ cōmixtū cui ſit acetum̄
Et bibitum̄ vermes ventris,tineaſqꝫ repellit
Ex oleo cum teſte ſua ſi decoquis illud
Morſus peſtiferos reddes hoc vnguine ſanos
Vnguine veſice dolor: ⁊ timor hoc reprimuntur
Corpus ⁊ attritum cura ſanabis eadem
Ipſe refert yppocras educi poſſe ſecundas
Fumo combuſti ſi vulua diu foueatur
Pulmonis varias coctum cum lacte querelas
Potatūqꝫ iuuat vel crudū ſepe comeſtum
Cum centaurea diodes dare precepit illud
Ydropicis,ſic humores deſiccat aquoſos
Idē nauſreticis elixum ſumere iuſſit
Pictagoras illo fuit vſus cum coriandro
Et vino cauſas ſic curans ictericorum
Et ſic potatum dicit ꝗ molliat aluum̄
Cunqꝫ faba coctū capitis ſedare dolorem